PET in CNS Disease

Guest Editors

ANDREW B. NEWBERG, MD
ABASS ALAVI, MD,
MD (Hon), PhD (Hon), DSc (Hon)

PET CLINICS

www.pet.theclinics.com

Consulting Editor
ABASS ALAVI, MD,
MD (Hon), PhD (Hon), DSc (Hon)

April 2010 • Volume 5 • Number 2

SAUNDERS an imprint of ELSEVIER, Inc.

W.B. SAUNDERS COMPANY
A Division of Elsevier Inc.

1600 John F. Kennedy Boulevard • Suite 1800 • Philadelphia, Pennsylvania 19103-2899

http://www.theclinics.com

PET CLINICS Volume 5, Number 2
April 2010 ISSN 1556-8598, ISBN-13: 978-1-4377-1942-0

Editor: Barton Dudlick

PET Clinics (ISSN 1556-8598) is published quarterly by Elsevier Inc., 360 Park Avenue South, New York, NY 10010-1710. Months of issue are January, April, July, and October. Periodicals postage paid at New York, NY, and additional mailing offices. Subscription prices per year are $196.00 (US individuals), $279.00 (US institutions), $97.00 (US students), $223.00 (Canadian individuals), $312.00 (Canadian institutions), $118.00 (Canadian students), $237.00 (foreign individuals), $312.00 (foreign institutions), and $118.00 (foreign students). To receive student and resident rate, orders must be accompanied by name of affiliated institution, date of term, and the signature of program/residency coordinator on institution letterhead. Orders will be billed at individual rate until proof of status is received. Foreign air speed delivery is included in all Clinics subscription prices. All prices are subject to change without notice. POSTMASTER: Send address changes to PET Clinics, Elsevier Health Sciences Division, Subscription Customer Service, 3251 Riverport Lane, Maryland Heights, MO 63043. **Customer Service: 1-800-654-2452 (U.S. and Canada); 314-447-8871 (outside U.S. and Canada). Fax: 314-447-8029. E-mail: journalscustomerservice-usa@elsevier.com (for print support); journalsonlinesupport-usa@elsevier.com (for online support).**

Reprints. For copies of 100 or more of articles in this publication, please contact the Commercial Reprints Department, Elsevier Inc., 360 Park Avenue South, New York, NY 10010-1710. Tel.: 212-633-3812; Fax: 212-462-1935; E-mail: reprints@elsevier.com.

Contributors

CONSULTING EDITOR

ABASS ALAVI, MD, MD (Hon), PhD (Hon), DSc (Hon)
Director of Research Education, Nuclear Medicine Section, Department of Radiology, Hospital of the University of Pennsylvania, Philadelphia, Pennsylvania

GUEST EDITORS

ANDREW B. NEWBERG, MD
Associate Professor, Division of Nuclear Medicine, Department of Radiology, Hospital of the University of Pennsylvania, Philadelphia, Pennsylvania

ABASS ALAVI, MD, MD (Hon), PhD (Hon), DSc (Hon)
Director of Research Education, Nuclear Medicine Section, Department of Radiology, Hospital of the University of Pennsylvania, Philadelphia, Pennsylvania

AUTHORS

ABASS ALAVI, MD, MD (Hon), PhD (Hon), DSc (Hon)
Director of Research Education, Nuclear Medicine Section, Department of Radiology, Hospital of the University of Pennsylvania, Philadelphia, Pennsylvania

FRÉDÉRIC ASSAL, MD
Neurology, Department of Clinical Neurosciences, Geneva University Hospital and Faculty of Medicine, Geneva, Switzerland

JACOB G. DUBROFF, MD, PhD
Division of Nuclear Medicine, Department of Radiology; Departments of Medicine and Neurology, Hospital of the University of Pennsylvania, Philadelphia, Pennsylvania

PACÔME FOSSE, MD
Division of Nuclear Medicine, University Hospital of Liège, University of Liège, Belgium

ROLAND HUSTINX, MD, PhD
Division of Nuclear Medicine, University Hospital of Liège, University of Liège, Belgium

ROBERT H. MACH, PhD
Professor, Department of Radiology, Mallinckrodt Institute of Radiology, Washington University School of Medicine, St. Louis, Missouri

MARIE-LOUISE MONTANDON, PhD
Division of Nuclear Medicine, Geneva University Hospital, Geneva, Switzerland

ANDREW B. NEWBERG, MD
Associate Professor, Division of Nuclear Medicine, Department of Radiology, Hospital of the University of Pennsylvania, Philadelphia, Pennsylvania

PAOLO NUCIFORA, MD, PhD
Assistant Professor, Department of Radiology, University of Pennsylvania, Philadelphia, Pennsylvania

SALLY W. SCHWARZ, MS, BCNP
Research Associate Professor, Department of Radiology, Mallinckrodt Institute of Radiology, Washington University School of Medicine, St. Louis, Missouri

HABIB ZAIDI, PhD, PD
Division of Nuclear Medicine, Geneva University Hospital; Geneva Neuroscience Center, Geneva University, Geneva, Switzerland

Contents

Preface ix

Andrew B. Newberg and Abass Alavi

Challenges for Developing PET Tracers: Isotopes, Chemistry, and Regulatory Aspects 131

Robert H. Mach and Sally W. Schwarz

The primary limitation on the development of new radiotracers for use with positron emission tomography (PET) is the time constraints created by working with radionuclides with the short half-lives inherent to carbon 11 and fluorine 18, the main radionuclides used in PET radiotracer development. In the past decade there have been several developments in the radiosynthetic methods used in PET chemistry, advances that are expected to lead to an increase in the number of radiotracers making the transition from clinical research studies to clinical PET studies. This article reviews developments in PET radiochemistry that will facilitate this process and discusses the application of these basic principles of PET radiotracer development in central nervous system research. Current status of regulatory requirements for the development of new PET radiotracers for imaging studies in humans is reviewed.

Structure-Function–Based Quantitative Brain Image Analysis 155

Habib Zaidi, Marie-Louise Montandon, and Frédéric Assal

Many neurodegenerative dementias produce significant alterations in the brain that are often not detectable by neurologic tests or with structural imaging. PET is ideally suited for monitoring cell/molecular events early in the course of a disease as well as during pharmacologic therapy. During the past 2 decades, molecular neuroimaging using PET and magnetic resonance (MR) has advanced elegantly and steadily gained importance in the clinical and research arenas. Software- and hardware-based multimodality brain imaging allowing the correlation between anatomic and molecular information has revolutionized clinical diagnosis and now offers unique capabilities for the clinical neuroimaging community and neuroscience researchers at large.

Evolving Role of Modern Structural and Functional MR Imaging Techniques for Assessing Neuropsychiatric Disorders 169

Paolo Nucifora

Structural and functional MR imaging techniques play an important role in the modern assessment of neuropsychiatric disorders. Applications of MR imaging are reviewed for several types of mental illness. Morphometric MR imaging, functional MR imaging, and diffusion tensor MR imaging all make unique contributions to the evolution of basic understanding, diagnosis, and treatment of mental illness.

PET in Brain Tumors 185

Roland Hustinx and Pacôme Fosse

Evaluating gliomas, either at diagnosis or at recurrence, is among the historical indications of FDG positron emission tomography (PET) imaging. There is a clear relationship between the tumor grade, patient prognosis, and intensity of uptake. Yet the exact role of FDG PET imaging remains debated. PET and methionine labeled with the short-lived C11 also have been proposed, with the significant advantage of high tumor-to-cortex contrast and distinct bological properties that lead to specific indications. Clinical use of this tracer is hampered by the need for an on-site cyclotron, however. In recent years, the increased availability of fluorinated amino-acid analogs, in particular FET, has open the way to renewed scientific interest in the field of neuro-oncological PET and PET/CT. This article discusses FDG and alternative tracers for diagnosing and characterizing primary brain tumors, detecting their recurrences, helping to guide the radiation therapy, and for evaluating the response to treatments.

PET Imaging for Traumatic Brain Injury **199**

Jacob G. Dubroff and Andrew B. Newberg

Traumatic brain injury represents a substantial public health problem for which clinicians have limited treatment avenues. Traditional FDG-positron emission tomography (PET) brain imaging has provided unique insights into this disease including prognostic information. With the advent and implementation of novel tracers as well as improvement in instrumentation, molecular brain imaging using PET can further illustrate traumatic brain injury pathophysiology and point to novel treatment strategies.

PET in Epilepsy and Other Seizure Disorders **209**

Abass Alavi and Andrew B. Newberg

Positron emission tomography (PET) imaging has been widely used in the evaluation and management of patients with seizure disorders. The ability of PET to measure cerebral function makes it ideal for studying the neurophysiologic correlates of seizure activity during ictal and interictal states. PET imaging is also useful for evaluating patients before surgical interventions to determine the best surgical method and maximize outcomes. Thus, PET will continue to play a major role not only in the clinical arena but in further investigations of the pathogenesis and management of various seizure disorders. This article reviews the literature regarding the current uses and indications for PET in the study and management of patients with seizure disorders.

Role of PET in the Investigation of Neuropsychiatric Disorders **223**

Andrew B. Newberg and Abass Alavi

PET imaging is used to assess a variety of psychiatric disorders. Most of these imaging results still lie in the realm of research, helping to understand the pathophysiology of different disorders, explore diagnostic criteria, and evaluate the effects of treatment. Future studies will be needed to explore how the growing number of neurotransmitter ligands can be used in the study of psychiatric disorders. Ultimately, identifying and validating clinical applications will be necessary so that PET imaging continues to play a key role in the management of psychiatric disorders.

Index **243**

PET Clinics

FORTHCOMING ISSUES

July 2010

Musculoskeletal PET
Roland Hustinx, MD,
Guest Editor

October 2010

Gynecologic Cancer
Ora Israel, MD,
Guest Editor

RECENT ISSUES

January 2010

PET Imaging of the Aging Brain
Andrew B. Newberg, MD, and
Abass Alavi, MD, *Guest Editors*

October 2009

Breast Cancer I
Sandip Basu, MD, Rakesh Kumar, MD,
Ayse Mavi, MD, and Abass Alavi, MD,
Guest Editors

RELATED INTEREST

July 2009
Seminars in Nuclear Medicine
Hybrid Imaging, Part I
Ora Israel, MD, and Martin Sandler, MD, *Guest Editors*

September 2009
Seminars in Nuclear Medicine
Hybrid Imaging, Part II
Ora Israel, MD, and Martin Sandler, MD, *Guest Editors*

GOAL STATEMENT
The goal of the *PET Clinics* is to keep practicing radiologists and radiology residents up to date with current clinical practice in positron emission tomography by providing timely articles reviewing the state of the art in patient care.

ACCREDITATION
PET Clinics is planned and implemented in accordance with the Essential Areas and Policies of the Accreditation Council for Continuing Medical Education (ACCME) through the joint sponsorship of the University of Virginia School of Medicine and Elsevier. The University of Virginia School of Medicine is accredited by the ACCME to provide continuing medical education for physicians.

The University of Virginia School of Medicine designates this educational activity for a maximum of 15 *AMA PRA Category 1 Credits*™ for each issue, 60 credits per year. Physicians should only claim credit commensurate with the extent of their participation in the activity.

The American Medical Association has determined that physicians not licensed in the US who participate in this CME activity are eligible for a maximum of 15 *AMA PRA Category 1 Credits*™ for each issue, 60 credits per year.

Category 1 credit can be earned by reading the text material, taking the CME examination online at http://www.theclinics.com/home/cme, and completing the evaluation. After taking the test, you will be required to review any and all incorrect answers. Following completion of the test and evaluation, your credit will be awarded and you may print your certificate.

FACULTY DISCLOSURE/CONFLICT OF INTEREST
The University of Virginia School of Medicine, as an ACCME accredited provider, endorses and strives to comply with the Accreditation Council for Continuing Medical Education (ACCME) Standards of Commercial Support, Commonwealth of Virginia statutes, University of Virginia policies and procedures, and associated federal and private regulations and guidelines on the need for disclosure and monitoring of proprietary and financial interests that may affect the scientific integrity and balance of content delivered in continuing medical education activities under our auspices.

The University of Virginia School of Medicine requires that all CME activities accredited through this institution be developed independently and be scientifically rigorous, balanced and objective in the presentation/discussion of its content, theories and practices.

All authors/editors participating in an accredited CME activity are expected to disclose to the readers relevant financial relationships with commercial entities occurring within the past 12 months (such as grants or research support, employee, consultant, stock holder, member of speakers bureau, etc.). The University of Virginia School of Medicine will employ appropriate mechanisms to resolve potential conflicts of interest to maintain the standards of fair and balanced education to the reader. Questions about specific strategies can be directed to the Office of Continuing Medical Education, University of Virginia School of Medicine, Charlottesville, Virginia.

The faculty and staff of the University of Virginia Office of Continuing Medical Education have no financial affiliations to disclose.

The authors/editors listed below have identified no professional or financial affiliations for themselves or their spouse/partner:

Abass Alavi, MD (Consulting Editor); Frédéric Assal, MD; Jacob G. Dubroff, MD, PhD; Barton Dudlick (Acquisitions Editor); Pacôme Fosse, MD; Roland Hustinx, MD, PhD; Marie-Louise Montandon, PhD; Andrew Newberg, MD (Guest Editor); Paolo Nucifora, MD, PhD; Patrice Rehm, MD (Test Author); and Habib Zaidi, PhD, PD.

The authors/editors listed below identified the following professional or financial affiliations for themselves or their spouse/partner:
Robert H. Mach, PhD is an industry funded research/investigator and has licensed patents with Isotrace Technologies.
Sally W. Schwarz, MS, BCNP is a consultant for Avid Radiopharmaceuticals.

Disclosure of Discussion of Non-FDA Approved Uses for Pharmaceutical Products and/or Medical Devices.
The University of Virginia School of Medicine, as an ACCME provider, requires that all faculty presenters identify and disclose any off-label uses for pharmaceutical and medical device products. The University of Virginia School of Medicine recommends that each physician fully review all the available data on new products or procedures prior to clinical use.

TO ENROLL
To enroll in the PET Clinics Continuing Medical Education program, call customer service at 1-800-654-2452 or visit us online at www.theclinics.com/home/cme. **The CME program is available to subscribers for an additional fee of $196.00.**

Preface

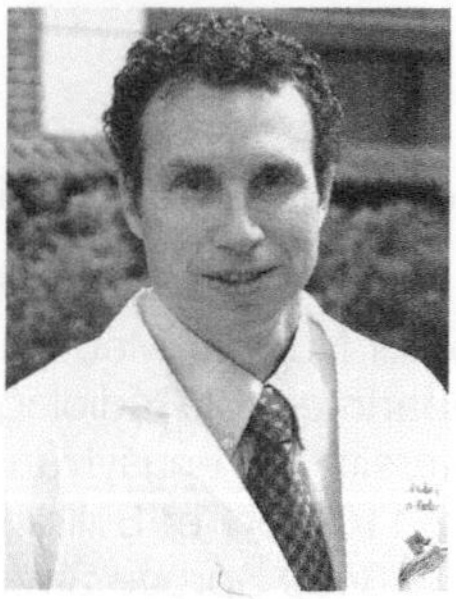
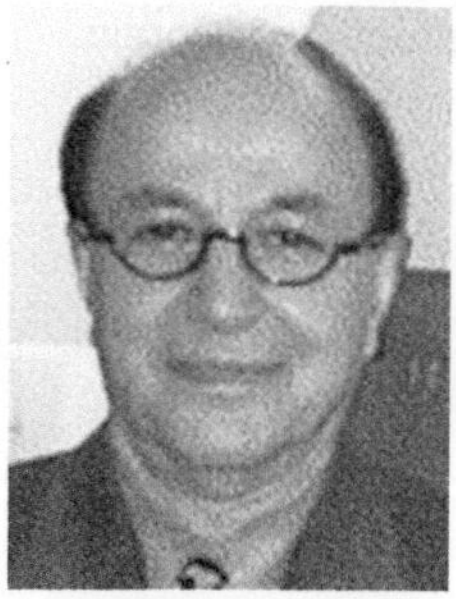

Andrew B. Newberg, MD   Abass Alavi, MD
Guest Editors

The use of PET has presented an important and unique opportunity for investigating neuropsychiatric disorders. PET imaging began with the development of ^{18}F-fluorodeoxyglucose (FDG) but has grown to include a multitude of radiopharmaceuticals that can evaluate almost any aspect of brain function. Emission tomography to image the biodistribution of radionuclides was originally developed in the 1960s by David Kuhl and Roy Edwards. This technique was later named single photon emission computed tomography (SPECT) and was used to study a number of neurologic disorders as well as to accurately demonstrate the regional distribution of various tracers in the central nervous system. SPECT studies use single photon-emitting radionuclides, such as iodine or technetium, that are labeled to a specific compound. Concurrent with these developments, it was realized that positron-emitting radionuclides allow for the synthesis of biologically important radiotracers because the elements used for labeling are identical or close to those that are naturally contained in such compounds. Thus, radionuclides, such as ^{11}C, ^{18}F, and ^{13}N, seem useful in producing a vast array of tracers that are optimal for studying the brain's chemistry and function. The emitted positron travels a short distance before meeting an electron and annihilating to produce 2 511-keV γ rays, which travel in opposite directions, approximately 180° from each other. Modern whole-body PET instruments have a resolution in the range of 3 to 4 mm. This resolution has approached the theoretic limit of a few millimeters, resulting in considerable improvement of image quality. Thus, PET is primed to be able to contribute substantially to the understanding of neuropsychiatric conditions in the future.

Over the past 35 years, PET imaging has been used to evaluate regional cerebral glucose metabolism in clinical and research applications. The array of disorders that has been studied include neurologic disorders, such as dementia, stroke, brain tumors, movement disorders, and seizures, and psychiatric disorders, including schizophrenia, mood disorders, anxiety, and drug abuse. One major development, which revealed the ability of PET to elucidate regional brain metabolism and function, was the synthesis of FDG. The early work performed with FDG PET had explored the metabolic landscape and changes associated with various neuropsychiatric disorders. This greatly advanced understanding of these disorders and the particular brain structures affected. More recent work has focused more on clinical issues, including diagnosis, management, and follow-up. Studies have also attempted to ascertain predictors of response to therapeutic interventions and have explored how specific activation paradigms might help uncover specific deficits not apparent with resting images.

Over this same period of time, a wide array of radiopharmaceuticals has been developed.

PET Clin 5 (2010) ix–x
doi:10.1016/j.cpet.2010.03.005
1556-8598/10/$ – see front matter

Tracers that can evaluate pre- and postsynaptic receptor function have been used to explore the dopamine, serotonin, glutamate, benzodiazepine, and opiate receptor systems. In addition, newer tracers have been developed that evaluate other pathophysiologic processes, such as amyloid deposition, hypoxia, and apoptosis. Each of these new tracers may have a variety of uses in the study of neuropsychiatric conditions.

The January and April issues of *PET Clinics* explore what PET imaging has revealed in a variety of neuropsychiatric disorders in the research and clinical settings. The articles describe the current status of PET data in different disorders, reveal current progress in understanding these disorders, and provide a foundation for future studies. It is important to show this overall perspective so that PET imaging can continue to be a highly valuable tool in the study of brain and the disorders affecting the brain.

Andrew B. Newberg, MD

Abass Alavi, MD
Division of Nuclear Medicine
Department of Radiology
Hospital of the University of Pennsylvania
110 Donner Building
3400 Spruce Street
Philadelphia, PA 19104, USA

E-mail addresses:
Andrew.newberg@uphs.upenn.edu (A.B. Newberg)
abass.alavi@uphs.upenn.edu (A. Alavi)

Challenges for Developing PET Tracers: Isotopes, Chemistry, and Regulatory Aspects

Robert H. Mach, PhD*, Sally W. Schwarz, MS, BCNP

KEYWORDS

• Carbon 11 • Fluorine 18 • PET regulatory • Chemistry

PET continues to be the primary functional imaging technique for conducting translational research studies aimed at identifying the molecular basis of human disease. Although PET imaging studies of the central nervous system (CNS) initially focused on global or regional changes in brain function such as glucose utilization, cerebral blood flow, and oxygen metabolism, a major effort in PET research in the past 20 years has focused on the development of specific probes that are capable of studying the change in neurotransmitter receptors, second messenger systems, and neuronal networks in the brain. As our knowledge of the diversity of neurotransmitter systems continues to grow, so will the need to develop molecular imaging probes with an even higher target specificity than first-generation PET radiotracers. For example, before the cloning of dopamine receptors, when PET imaging studies of the dopamine D_2 receptor began in the mid-1980s, it was believed that there were only 2 types of dopamine receptors: D_1 and D_2. It is now known that there are 2 different families of dopamine receptors: D_1-like (consisting of the D_1 and D_5 receptors) and D_2-like (consisting of the D_2, D_3, and D_4 receptors).[1] There is a growing body of evidence that within the D_2-like family of receptors, D_2 and D_3 receptors are regulated in an opposing manner under conditions of increased or decreased dopaminergic tone. For example, autoradiography studies have shown that there is a 15% increase in D_2 receptors in the caudate and putamen and a 45% decrease in D_3 receptors in the ventral striatum of postmortem brain samples of Parkinson disease.[2] Similar results have been reported in the study of chronic exposure to cocaine on D_2 and D_3 receptor function. That is, D_2 receptors are reduced in autoradiography[3] and PET imaging studies of rhesus monkeys that have self-administered cocaine,[4] and in chronic cocaine abusers.[5,6] However, the autoradiography studies conducted by Staley and Mash[7] reported an upregulation of D_3 receptors in human cocaine overdose victims compared with age-matched controls. Because PET radiotracers such as $[^{11}C]$raclopride, $[^{18}F]$fallypride, and $[^{11}C]$PHNO have a high affinity for D_2 and D_3 receptors, newer radiotracers having a higher affinity and selectivity for D_3 versus D_2 receptors are needed to study the role of the D_3 receptor in CNS disorders. This same argument can be applied to many other CNS receptor systems, including the serotonergic system (7 different families for receptors and at least 13 different receptor subtypes),[8] glutamate receptors (2 different classes, ionic and metabotropic, with at least 11 different subtypes),[9] and the adrenergic receptors (6 different subtypes of α adrenergic receptors and 3 different subtypes of β receptors).[10] As the need for more subtype-selective radiotracers grows, the success criteria for these newer radiotracers are expected to be higher than PET chemists have

Department of Radiology, Mallinckrodt Institute of Radiology, Washington University School of Medicine, 510 South Kingshighway Boulevard, St Louis, MO 63110, USA
* Corresponding author.
E-mail address: rhmach@mir.wustl.edu

PET Clin 5 (2010) 131–153
doi:10.1016/j.cpet.2010.02.002

striven to achieve in the past. For example, as a PET radiotracer becomes more subtype selective, the target density to be imaged by the tracer within the CNS (ie, receptor density or B_{max}) invariably decreases. The development of high-affinity, high-selectivity, and low-nonspecific-binding radiotracers will likely be required to provide a suitable signal-to-noise ratio in PET imaging studies. Factors such as improved specific activity also play a key role in the ability to image receptors, and other protein targets that have a low expression in the CNS.

This article does not review the advances in radiotracer design with respect to subtype-selective PET imaging probes; that topic is covered in other articles in this and other issues of *PET Clinics*. This article provides an overview of the basic principles of PET radiochemistry and describes recent advances in PET radiosynthesis to assist the development of subtype-selective PET radiotracers needed to address the next level of scientific inquiry within clinical neuroscience research. The general principles of radiotracer design used by many chemists in the development of a PET radiotracer are also described, especially when this involves the incorporation of fluorine 18 (^{18}F) into a molecule that does not possess a fluorine atom. A description of the current regulatory guidelines relevant to the production of PET radiotracers for human use studies is also provided.

RADIONUCLIDES USED IN PET

The 4 positron-emitting radionuclides most frequently used in PET are oxygen 15 (^{15}O), nitrogen 13 (^{13}N), carbon 11 (^{11}C), and ^{18}F. There are several reasons why these radionuclides are routinely used in PET imaging applications. The first is that most of these radionuclides can be substituted into biologically active molecules with a hot-for-cold substitution. That is, ^{11}C can be substituted for nonradioactive ^{12}C in a biologically active molecule without altering the biologic properties of the molecule. In this example, ^{11}C is a true radiotracer because the structure of the biologically active molecule has not been altered to introduce the PET radiolabel. The same concept applies to ^{15}O and ^{13}N; however, the short half-lives of ^{15}O and ^{13}N have limited their use in PET radiotracer development. Consequently, these radionuclides are largely used as perfusion tracers: [^{15}O]water for brain perfusion studies and [^{13}N]ammonia for heart perfusion studies.

An exception to the principle of hot-for-cold substitution is ^{18}F; although fluorine is the most abundant halogen in soil samples, the abundance of naturally occurring organofluorine compounds is low and limited to fluorinated carboxylic acids such as fluoroacetate, fluorocitrate, and fluorinated fatty acids produced in numerous plant species indigenous to Africa, Australia, and South America.[11] There are no naturally occurring organofluorine compounds in animals. However, fluorine is a frequently used substituent in drug development, and there are several fluorine-containing drugs targeting neurotransmitter receptors in the CNS.[12] These include the antidepressants fluoxetine and paroxetine, the tricyclic antipsychotic fluphenazine, the butyrophenones haloperidol and spiperone, and the atypical antipsychotics risperidone and setoperone. These fluorine-containing drugs have served as a direct source of leads for PET radiotracers involving the principle of an ^{18}F for ^{19}F substitution.[13–19] In addition to these examples, it is often possible to incorporate fluorine into a nonfluorine-containing lead compound without losing activity at the target protein; 1 example is the dopamine D_2 imaging agent fluoroclebopride, an analogue of the dopamine antagonist clepopride.[20]

A second reason for the prominent use of these radionuclides in PET imaging studies is that each can be produced in high yield and high specific activity with a low energy (ie, 11–17 MeV), medical cyclotron using either the p,n (^{15}O, ^{13}N, ^{18}F) or p,α (^{11}C) nuclear reaction (**Table 1**). Because the

Table 1
Radionuclides commonly used in PET

Radionuclide	Half-life (min)	Nuclear Reaction	Average β + Energy (keV)	β + Range mm (H_2O)	Maximum Specific Activity (Ci/μmol)
Oxygen 15	2	$^{15}N(p,n)^{15}O$	735	8.2	91730
Nitrogen 13	10	$^{13}C(p,n)^{13}N$	491	5.39	18900
Carbon 11	20	$^{14}N(p,\alpha)^{11}C$	385	4.1	9220
Fluorine 18	110	$^{18}O(p,n)^{18}F$	242	2.39	1710

Routine specific activity: ^{11}C, ~10 Ci/μmol; [^{18}F]fluoride, 2–10 Ci/μmol.

target material is either gas (^{15}O, ^{11}C) or liquid (^{13}N, ^{18}F), the radionuclides are readily transferred from the cyclotron target to a hot cell in the radiochemistry laboratory, where the radionuclide can be incorporated into a biologically active molecule. There are also several commercially available automated chemistry systems that are capable of converting these PET radionuclides, obtained as low molecular weight species from the cyclotron target, into either a chemically reactive species or a radiolabeled prosthetic group. Automated chemistry systems are typically designed to conduct 2 to 3 organic reactions in series, followed by either a resin-based or high-performance liquid chromatography (HPLC) purification step, leading to the synthesis of a PET radiotracer that is suitable for imaging studies in preclinical imaging studies in animal models or in clinical research studies. Although simplistic in theory, the adaptation of a commercially available automated PET chemistry system to enable the synthesis of structurally diverse PET radiotracers, and the routine review and optimization of the synthesis to ensure reproducible radiochemical yields and high specific activity, requires considerable expertise in organic chemistry and chemical engineering. Quality assurance testing to confirm that the radiotracer meets criteria for radiochemical and chemical purity, specific activity, sterility, pyrogen levels, and presence of residual solvents for use in humans also requires expertise in analytical chemistry and radiopharmacy. Therefore, most PET centers actively engaged in clinical research consist of a collaboration between organic/medicinal chemists, chemical engineers, analytical chemists, and radiopharmacists working in concert to meet the significant time constraints imposed by the short-lived radioisotopes routinely used in PET.

Because ^{11}C and ^{18}F are the 2 main radionuclides used in the development of PET radiotracers for imaging brain function, this article focuses on a review of the basic principles and recent developments in the radiosynthesis of ^{11}C- and ^{18}F-labeled compounds.

^{11}C Radiochemistry

^{11}C is produced in the cyclotron target using the $^{14}N(p,\alpha)^{11}C$ nuclear reaction. The target material is nitrogen (N_2) containing trace quantities of oxygen (0.5% O_2) to convert the ^{11}C into [^{11}C]CO_2.[21,22] The simplest reaction using ^{11}C involves the transfer of [^{11}C]CO_2 from the target to a chemistry module or a reaction vessel containing a Grignard reagent that reacts with [^{11}C]CO_2 to give the corresponding ^{11}C-labeled carboxylic acid. The most prominent examples of this process are the metabolic tracers [^{11}C]acetate and [^{11}C]palmitate (**Fig. 1**), which are prepared by the direct venting of [^{11}C]CO_2 into a solution of either methylmagnesium bromide or 1-pentadecylmagnesium bromide in an anhydrous solvent such as tetrahydrofuran or ether.[23] There are 2 examples in which [^{11}C]CO_2 has been used in the synthesis of a PET radiotracer for imaging CNS receptors: (1) the serotonin 5-hydroxytryptamine$_{1A}$ (5-HT$_{1A}$) antagonist [^{11}C]Way-10065[24,25]; and (2) the radiolabeled dopamine D_2/D_3 agonist, [^{11}C](+)-PHNO, which is primarily used to image the high affinity state of the dopamine D_2 and D_3 receptors.[26–28] In each case, [^{11}C]CO_2 is vented through a solution of the Grignard reagent (cyclohexyl magnesium chloride for Way-10065 and ethylmagnesium bromide for (+)-PHNO) to give ^{11}C-labeled carboxylic acid; conversion to the corresponding acid chloride results in the formation of ^{11}C-labeled acid chloride, which is reacted with the secondary amine (see **Fig. 1**) to give the corresponding amide. Synthesis of [^{11}C](+)-PHNO requires the additional reduction of the amide with lithium aluminum hydride resulting in the formation of [^{11}C](+)-PHNO.[26]

The most common chemical transformation of [^{11}C]CO_2 is into [^{11}C]methyliodide ([^{11}C]CH_3I) (**Fig. 2**), a highly reactive species that can be used to introduce ^{11}C into biologically active molecules via alkylation of N-, O-, or S-nucleophiles (**Fig. 3**). The initial method for preparing [^{11}C]CH_3I involved passing [^{11}C]CO_2 through a solution of lithium aluminum hydride ($LiAlH_4$) and tetrahydrofuran (see **Fig. 3**), followed by quenching with hydrioidic acid. This method has been largely replaced with the gas phase method of synthesizing [^{11}C]methyl iodide, which involves the catalytic reduction of [^{11}C]CO_2 to [^{11}C]methane ([^{11}C]CH_4), followed by iodination with molecular iodine (I_2) to produce [^{11}C]CH_3I. An alternative method for preparing [^{11}C]CH_3I involves the direct production of [^{11}C]CH_4 by using a target gas composition of 10% H_2/N_2 in the target, followed by iodination with molecular I_2 (see **Fig. 2**). The rationale for using the in-target production of [^{11}C]CH_4 is the lower amount of methane in the atmosphere (~1.6 ppm) relative to CO_2 (~300 ppm); in theory, this should result in improved specific activity of [^{11}C]CH_3I. However, the inexplicable low recovery for the in-target production of [^{11}C]CH_4 has prevented the widespread use of this method for the synthesis of [^{11}C]CH_3I. Average specific activities of ^{11}C-labeled radiotracers using [^{11}C]CH_3I have been reported in the range of 2 to 10 Ci/μmol (74–370 GBq/μmol). This specific activity is lower than the

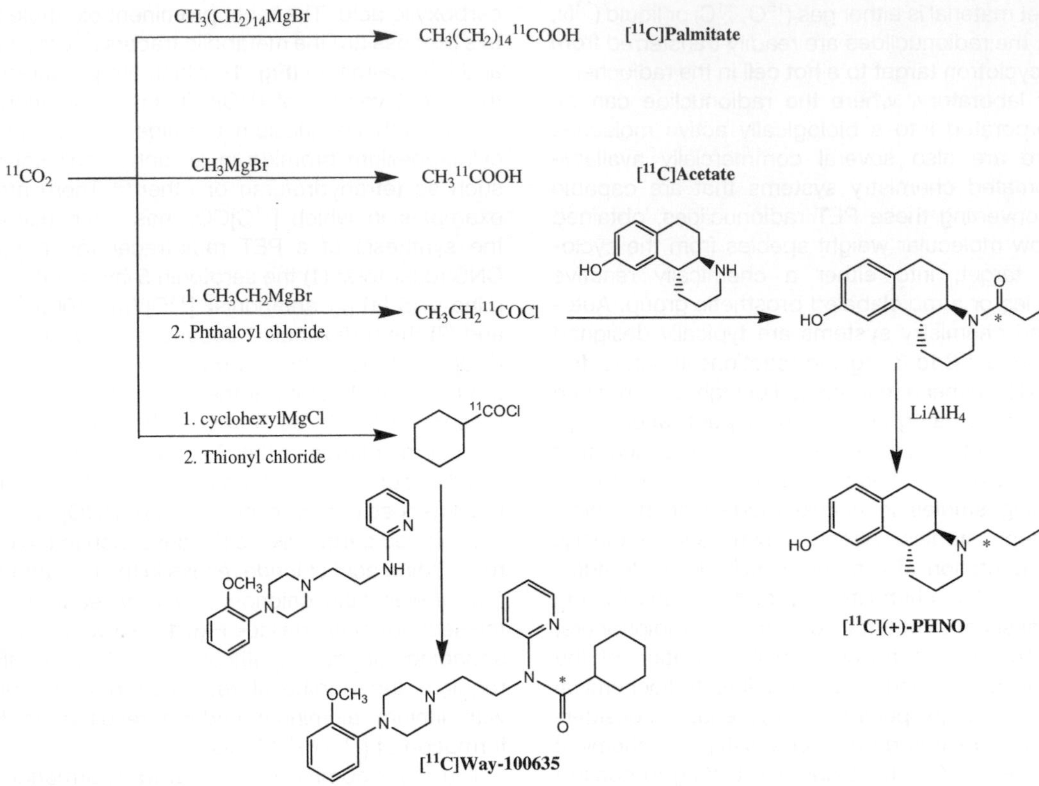

Fig. 1. Synthesis of [^{11}C]palmitate, [^{11}C]acetate, [^{11}C](+)-PHNO and [^{11}C]Way-100635 using [^{11}C]CO_2.

maximum theoretic specific activity of ^{11}C (see **Table 1**). Therefore, for an ^{11}C-labeled radiotracer having a specific activity of 10 Ci/mmol, only 1 in 1000 tracer molecules contain ^{11}C, with the remaining containing ^{12}C.

Another highly reactive form of ^{11}C is [^{11}C]methyltriflate ([^{11}C]CH_3OTf). [^{11}C]CH_3OTf is formed by passing gaseous [^{11}C]CH_3I over a column containing silver triflate (AgOTf) at 200°C (see **Fig. 2**).[21] The advantage of [^{11}C]CH_3OTf is that this method generally requires lower reaction temperatures, shorter reaction times, and lower amounts of the *des*-methyl precursor for labeling than is usually required to label a compound using [^{11}C]CH_3I. Because HPLC retention times of the *des*-methyl precursor are similar to the ^{11}C-labeled *N*-methyl product, reducing the amount of precursor for the labeling reaction can simplify the HPLC purification of the radiotracer as a result of a reduced tendency of peak broadening by the *des*-methyl precursor. Although this time saving may seem trivial, reducing the synthesis time from 30 minutes to 25 minutes leads to an approximately 20% increase in specific activity of a ^{11}C-labeled radiotracer simply by reducing the loss of activity by radioactive decay. Examples comparing radiolabeling with [^{11}C]CH_3I and [^{11}C]CH_3OTf are shown in **Fig. 4**.[22,29–31] Perhaps the best example of the advantage of [^{11}C]CH_3OTf over [^{11}C]CH_3I is the synthesis of the β amyloid imaging agent [^{11}C]PiB. The synthesis of [^{11}C]PiB from [^{11}C]CH_3I requires the addition of a base such as

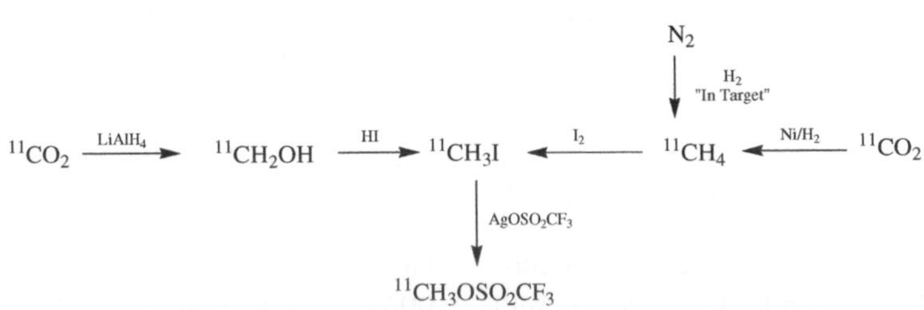

Fig. 2. Synthesis of [^{11}C]CH_3I and [^{11}C]CH_3OTf.

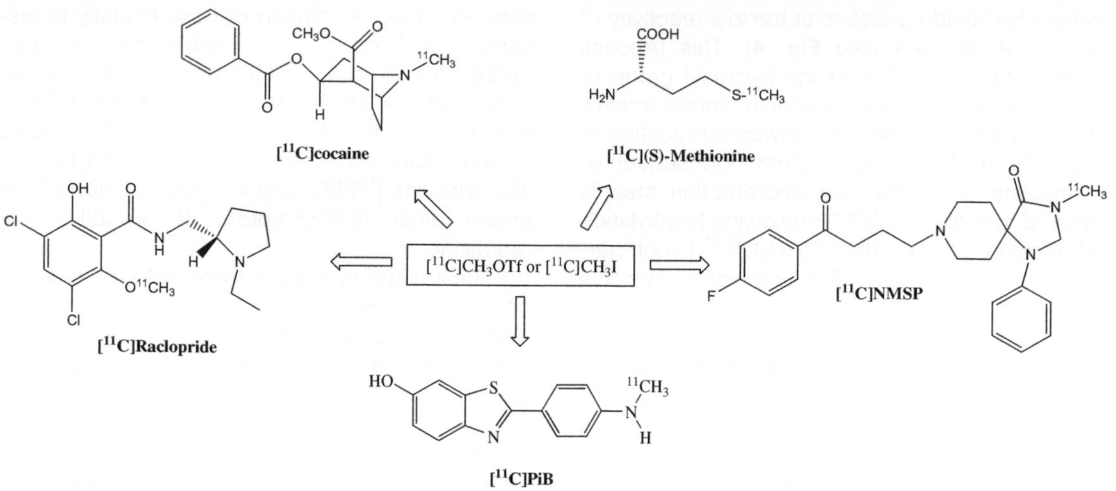

Fig. 3. Examples of ^{11}C-labeled radiotracers synthesized using [^{11}C]CH_3I or [^{11}C]CH_3OTf.

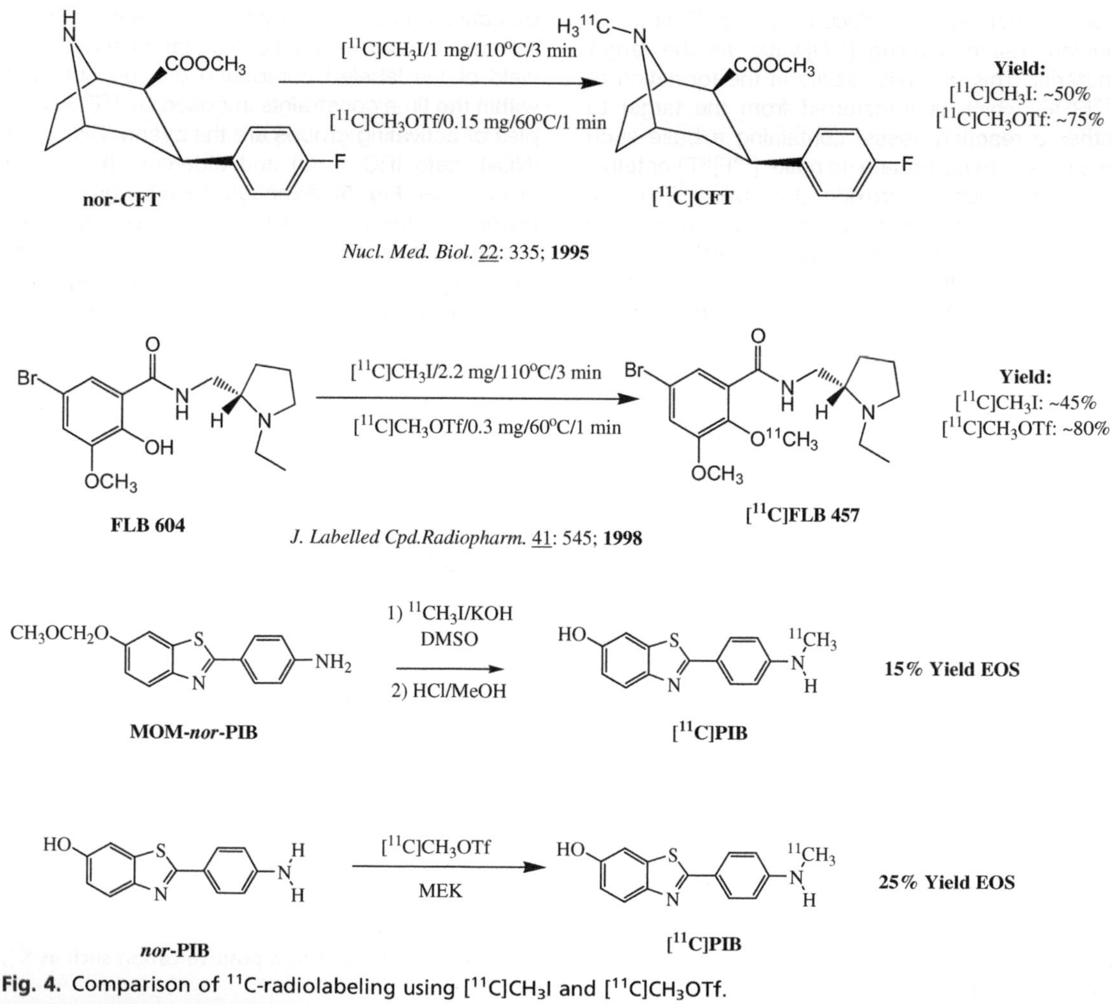

Fig. 4. Comparison of ^{11}C-radiolabeling using [^{11}C]CH_3I and [^{11}C]CH_3OTf.

sodium hydroxide because of the low reactivity of the amine nitrogen (see **Fig. 4**). This process requires the protection of the hydroxyl group of the precursor as the corresponding methoxymethyl (MOM) ether to prevent the unwanted reaction of [^{11}C]CH_3I at the oxygen atom. Consequently, a separate acid-catalyzed deprotection step is required to prepare [^{11}C]PiB following N-alkylation of the amine group with [^{11}C]CH_3I.[32,33] In comparison, because [^{11}C]CH_3OTf has a higher chemical reactivity than [^{11}C]CH_3I, the reaction at the aniline nitrogen occurs without the addition of a base catalyst, thereby eliminating the need to protect the phenol group as the corresponding MOM ether. This 1-step synthesis using [^{11}C]CH_3OTf is the preferred method for making [^{11}C]PiB because of its shorter synthesis time and higher radiochemical yield.[34–36]

^{18}F Radiochemistry

Two forms of ^{18}F are used in the synthesis of PET radiotracers: nucleophilic and electrophilic. Nucleophilic fluoride is produced via the ^{18}O(p,n)^{18}F nuclear reaction using [^{18}O]water as the target material. This process results in the formation of [^{18}F]HF, which is transferred from the target to either a reaction vessel containing a base such as potassium carbonate (to make [^{18}F]KF) or tetrabutylammonium hydroxide (to give [^{18}F]TBAF). Alternatively, the radioactivity can be passed through an anion exchange resin, which traps the activity as [^{18}F]fluoride. The activity is then removed from the anion exchange resin by elution with an aqueous solution of base (usually potassium carbonate or tetrabutylammonium hydroxide) to give [^{18}F]fluoride as a salt (ie, [^{18}F]KF or [^{18}F]TBAF). An advantage of [^{18}F]TBAF is that it can be directly solubilized into organic solvents such as acetonitrile and dimethylsulfoxide, whereas [^{18}F]KF requires the addition of the crown ether [2.2.2]kryptofix to solubilize the reactivity.

[^{18}F]Fluoride is incorporated into biologically active molecules via 2 types of reaction mechanisms: SN2 and SNAr2. The SN2 mechanism occurs when an appropriate leaving group is displaced from an aliphatic (ie, sp3) carbon atom (**Fig. 5**). The SNAr2 mechanism occurs when the leaving group is displaced from an aromatic (ie, sp2) carbon atom such as a benzene ring. Although fluoride is a relatively unreactive nucleophile, high yields of an ^{18}F-labeled radiotracer can be obtained with the SN2 mechanism if the precursor contains a good leaving group such as a triflate (R = CF_3) or mesylate (R = CH_3) group. In the SNAr2 mechanism, the para position must be activated by an electron-withdrawing group to increase the rate of reaction so that an acceptable yield of the labeled compound can be obtained within the time constraints imposed by ^{18}F. Examples of activating groups are the cyano (CN), nitro (NO_2), keto (RC = O) and aldehyde (HC = O) groups (see **Fig. 5**). Although the nitro group was historically the first leaving group used in radiofluorinations using the SNAr2 mechanism, the trimethylammonium group is more commonly used today because of its rapid rate of reaction and

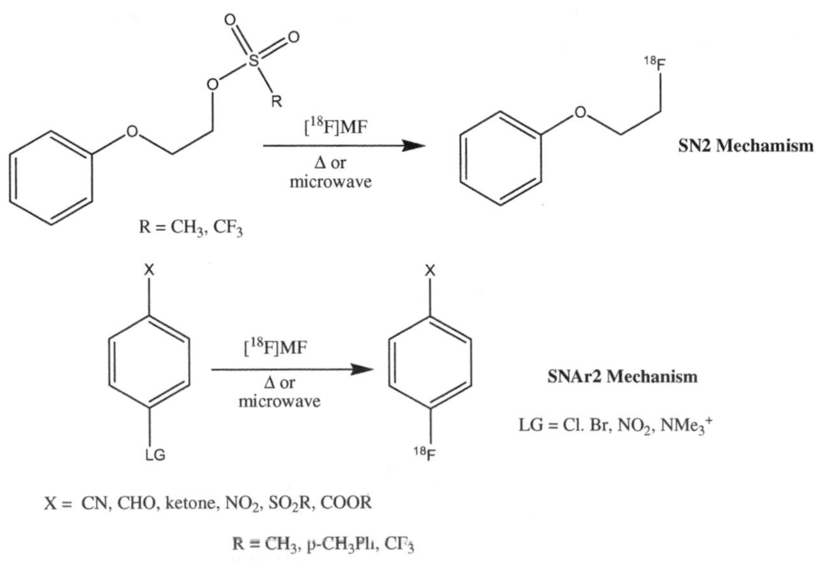

Fig. 5. Reaction mechanism for introducing ^{18}F into organic molecules. M refers to a positive cation such as K^+, Cs^+, or $(Bu)_4N^+$.

the ease of eliminating unreacted precursor resulting from the high polarity of the charged trimethylammonium group.[37] There are 2 methods used for increasing the rate of reactivity of [^{18}F]fluoride: heating the reaction mixture (from 90 to 160 °C) and microwave irradiation. Microwave irradiation is rapidly becoming the preferred method of nucleophilic [^{18}F]fluoride incorporation because the reaction time needed to achieve a high radiochemical yield of the product is typically faster than the simple thermal method of incorporation.

Although activation of the paraposition within 1 of these groups facilitates the incorporation of [^{18}F]fluoride, it does not guarantee a high radiochemical yield. An example of this is shown in **Fig. 6**. Whereas [^{18}F]fluoride is readily incorporated into the nitroprecursor, resulting in a high radiochemical yield of [^{18}F]setoperone, similar reaction conditions result in only a low yield of [^{18}F]*N*-methylspiperone even although both substrates have a ketone as the activating group in the paraposition.[19,38] The low yield of [^{18}F]*N*-methylspiperone is likely caused by keto-enol tautomerization, which leads to the formation of the nonreactive enol (see **Fig. 6**). Because of the long half-life of ^{18}F (110 minutes), a multistep synthesis of [^{18}F]NMSP was developed[39] (**Fig. 7**), which afforded yields suitable for human imaging studies.[40]

A second example of the SNAr2 reaction mechanism for incorporating ^{18}F into biologically active molecules involves the displacement of a leaving group in either the 2 or 6 position of a pyridine ring. Because pyridine is a π-deficient heteroaromatic ring system, it is prone to nucleophilic attack at the 2, 4, and 6 positions. Therefore, a pyridine ring does not require the presence of an electron-withdrawing group to activate the ring system to nucleophilic attack by [^{18}F]fluoride. This strategy has been used extensively in the synthesis of ligands for imaging nicotinic $\alpha_4\beta_2$ receptors (**Fig. 8**).[41–44]

An alternative strategy for introducing high specific activity, nucleophilic [^{18}F]fluoride into ligands is to use an ^{18}F-labeled prosthetic group. This method uses the same basic principle as labeling a molecule with [^{11}C]CH_3I, which is essentially an ^{11}C-labeled prosthetic group. In this approach, ^{18}F is incorporated into an organic molecule, which is then used to alkylate a precursor leading to an ^{18}F-labeled radiotracer.[17] As with [^{11}C]CH_3I, the most common reaction is the alkylation of a nitrogen atom. The following different ^{18}F-labeled prosthetic groups have been used to date: [^{18}F]2-fluoroethoxytriflate or [^{18}F]2-fluoroethyltosylate[45,46]; and, [^{18}F]4-fluorobenzyl iodide (or bromide).[47–49] Examples

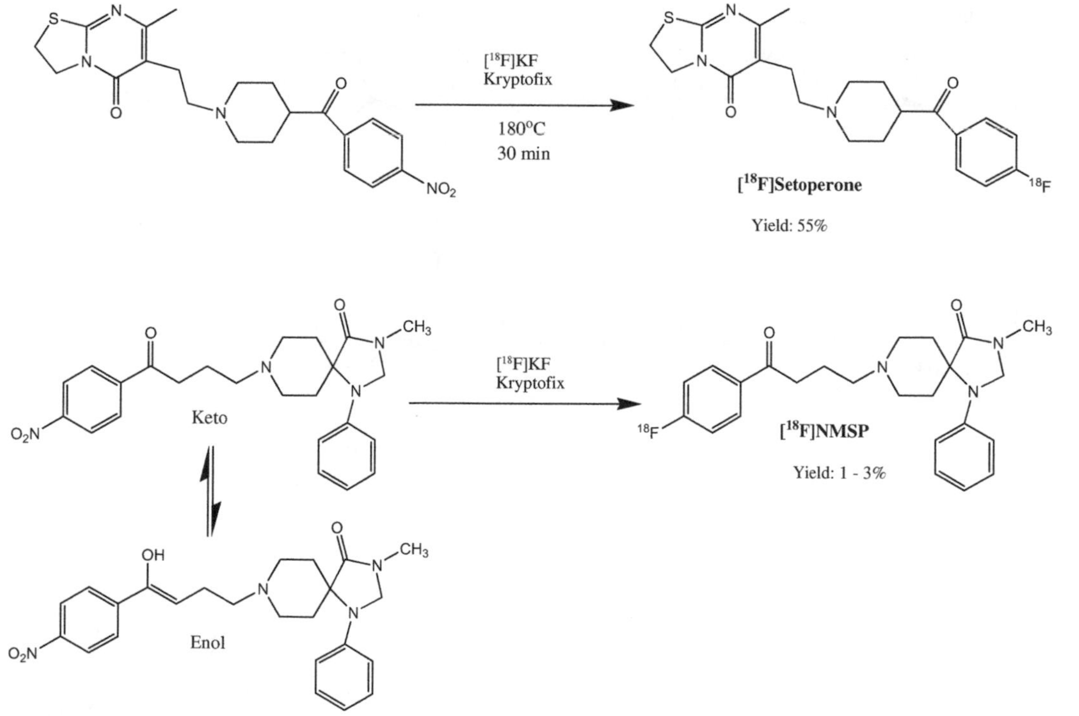

Fig. 6. Examples of nucleophilic incorporation of [^{18}F]fluoride. Note the difference in radiochemical yield even although both substrates are activated by a ketone group in the para position.

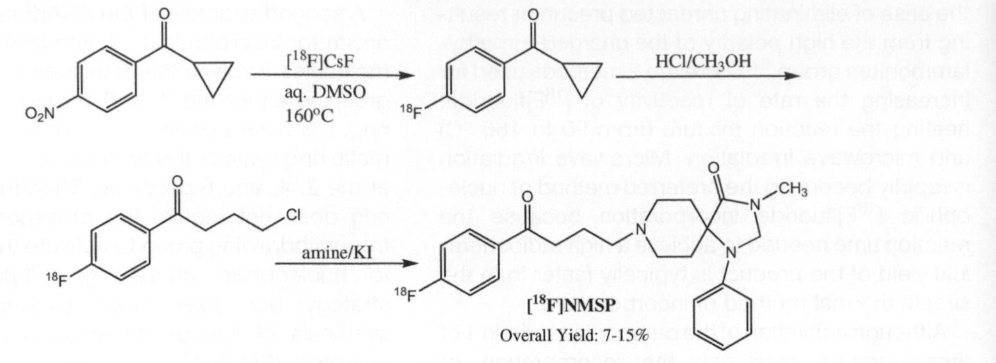

Fig. 7. Synthesis of [^{18}F]NMSP by the PET group at Brookhaven National Laboratory.

of the use of these prosthetic groups in radiotracer synthesis are shown in **Figs. 9** and **10**.

A recent development in PET radiochemistry is the use of copper-assisted 1,3-dipolar cycloaddition reactions to prepare ^{18}F-labeled compounds. The method, often referred to as click chemistry, uses either an ^{18}F-labeled fluorinated acetylene or an ^{18}F-labeled organic azide as the prosthetic group (**Fig. 11**). The first click radiolabeling reactions used simple [^{18}F]fluoroalkynes[50] and [^{18}F]2-fluoroethylazide.[51] Reported radiochemical yield using this strategy has been high, often in excess of 80%.[50,51] This labeling strategy has been used most often in the radiolabeling of peptides because it avoids the need to protect the multiple functional groups in a polypeptide that could react with the prosthetic groups currently used in producing ^{18}F-labeled peptides (**Fig. 12**). Several second-generation ^{18}F-labeled click synthons have been introduced recently[52–54] and are shown in **Fig. 11**. A review of the use of click chemistry in PET radiotracer design was recently published by Glaser and Robbins.[55]

A second method for introducing ^{18}F into biologically active molecules is through the use of an electrophilic fluorination reaction with [^{18}F]F_2.

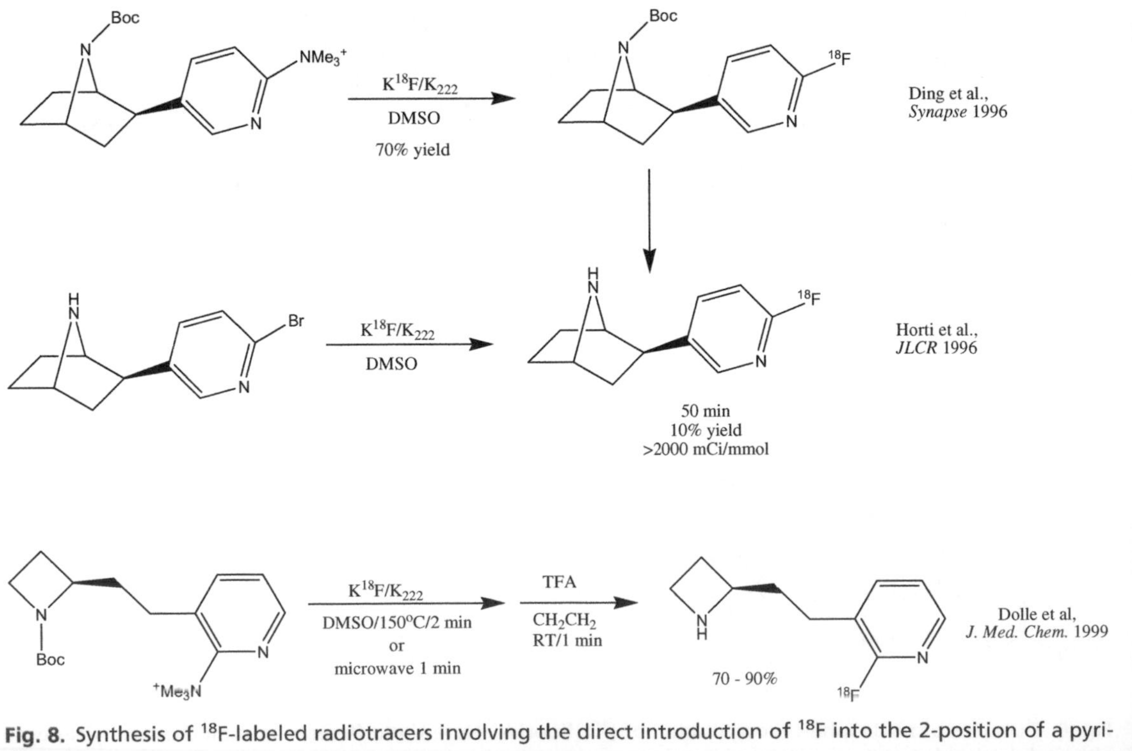

Fig. 8. Synthesis of ^{18}F-labeled radiotracers involving the direct introduction of ^{18}F into the 2-position of a pyridine ring.

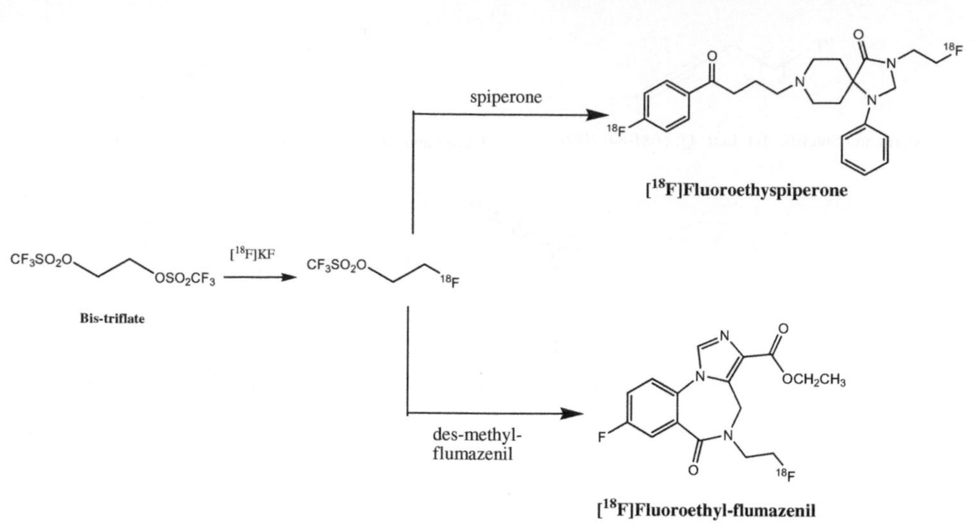

Fig. 9. Radiosynthesis using the [^{18}F]2-fluoroethoxytriflate as a prosthetic group.

There are 2 different ways to produce electrophilic [^{18}F]F_2. The first method, which requires a cyclotron designed to accelerate deuterons, is the ^{20}Ne(d,α)^{18}F nuclear reaction (**Fig. 13**). The neon target gas contains ~2% F_2 to complete the in-target production of [^{18}F]F_2. The second method for producing [^{18}F]F_2 involves the ^{18}O(p,n)^{18}F nuclear reaction. This method, which is generally used on proton-only cyclotrons, requires a multistep process to produce

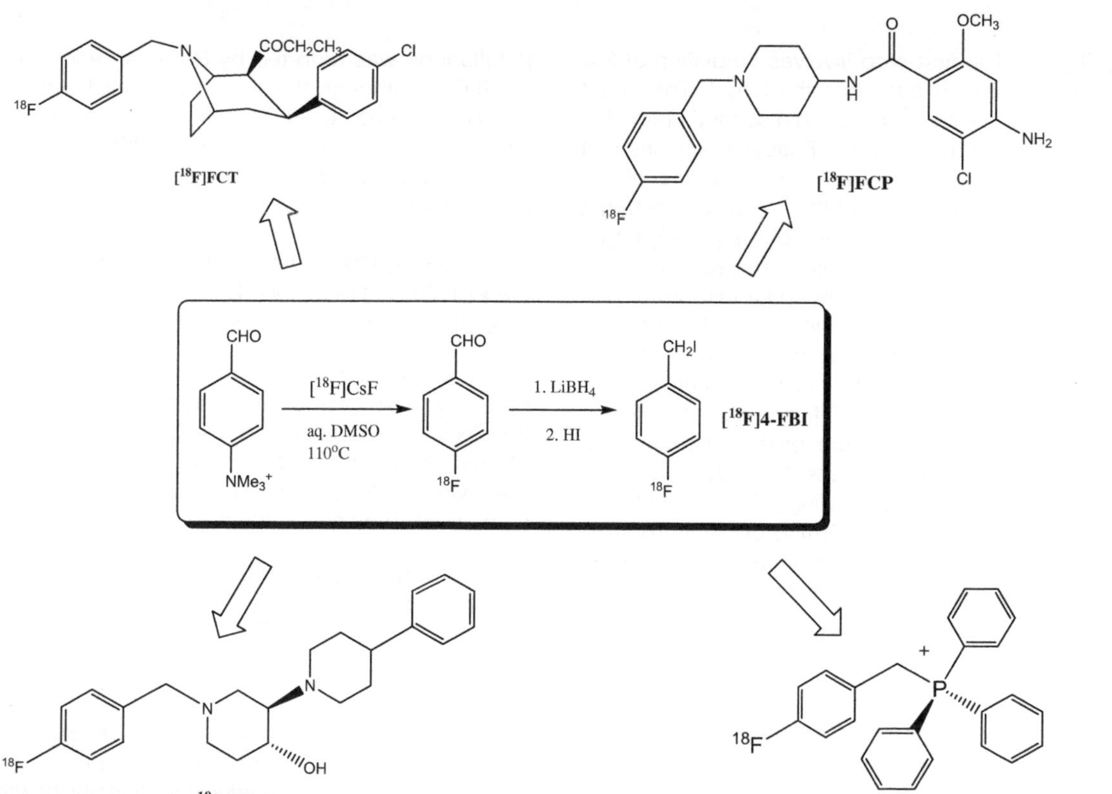

Fig. 10. Examples of ^{18}F radiolabeling using the prosthetic group, [^{18}F]4-fluorobenzyl iodide. (*Data from* Refs.[47–49])

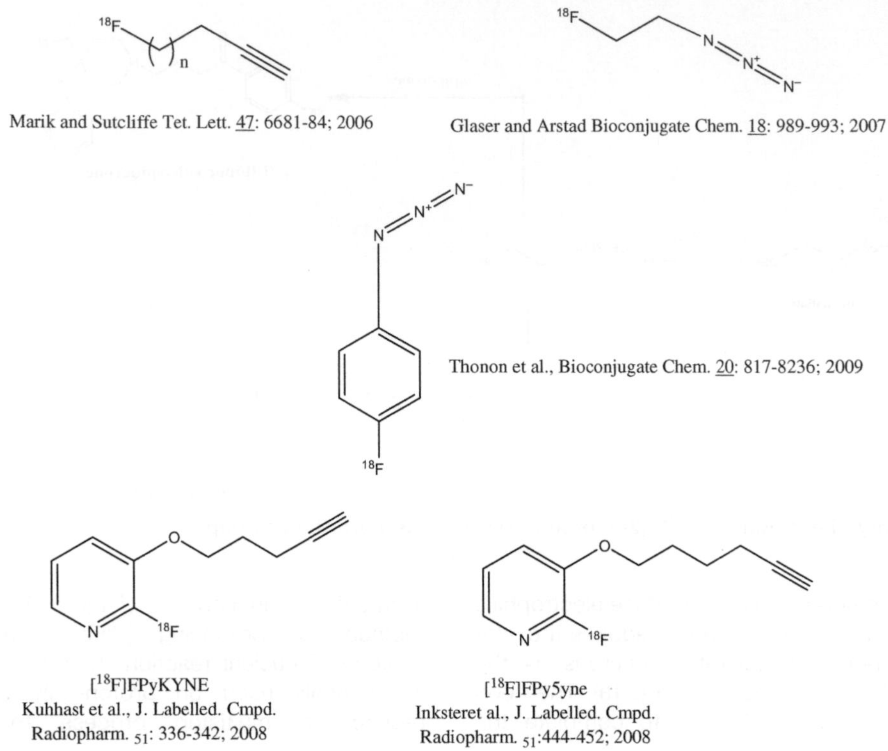

Fig. 11. Prosthetic groups used in click labeling with ^{18}F.

[^{18}F]F_2.[56] The first step involves irradiation of 2% F_2/Ar mixture to passivate the target. The target is then filled with [^{18}O]O_2, and a second irradiation is conducted to produce ^{18}F-labeled species that are deposited on to the interior surface of the target. This deposition of the ^{18}F on to the target surface enables the recovery of the [^{18}F]O_2 target gas. Once the [^{18}O]O_2 has been recovered, the target is filled with 2%F_2/Ar and a third irradiation is conducted to recover the [^{18}F]F_2. Electrophilic fluorination with [^{18}F]F_2 is the preferred method for making [^{18}F]fluoro-L-dihydroxyphenylalanine ([^{18}F]FDOPA)[57] and [^{18}F]fluoro-meta-tyrosine,[58] radiotracers that measure presynaptic dopaminergic terminal density (see **Fig. 13**). Other PET radiotracer synthesized using [^{18}F]F_2 include 2β-carbomethoxy-3β-(4-[^{18}F]-fluorophenyl)tropane, [^{18}F]CFT,[59] which labels the dopamine transporter (another marker of dopamine terminal density) and 2-(2-nitro-^{1}H-imidazol-1-yl)-N-(2,2,3,3,3-pentafluoropropyl)-acetamide (EF-5) labeled with ^{18}F-fluorine, [^{18}F]EF-5, a radiotracer for imaging hypoxia.[60] The main drawback to using electrophilic fluorination for introducing ^{18}F is low specific activity that is achieved using [^{18}F]F_2, because of the requirement of adding unlabeled F_2 to recover the radioactivity from the target. However, a method for producing electrophilic [^{18}F]F_2 from nucleophilic [^{18}F]fluoride was reported by Bergman and Solin in 1997.[61] Although the addition of unlabeled F_2 is still required to form [^{18}F]F_2, a significant increase in specific activity of [^{18}F]FDOPA and [^{18}F]CFT have been reported using this method of electrophilic radiofluorination.[61]

FACTORS DETERMINING THE ABILITY OF PET RADIOTRACERS TO CROSS THE BLOOD-BRAIN BARRIER

There are several factors to contend with in the design of a radiotracer for imaging targets within the CNS. A description of these factors of prerequisites for CNS PET radiotracers can be found in the review by Ametamey and colleagues.[62] A brief summary is provided in the next section.

Affinity and Selectivity for the Target Receptor or Enzyme

Ideally, a PET probe should possess a high (ie, nanomolar) affinity and high selectivity (>100-fold) for the target protein versus other proteins in the CNS. However, the exact affinity of a suitable PET ligand for its target protein depends on a variety of factors, including the density of the receptor or protein target, the presence of endogenous ligands that could compete with the

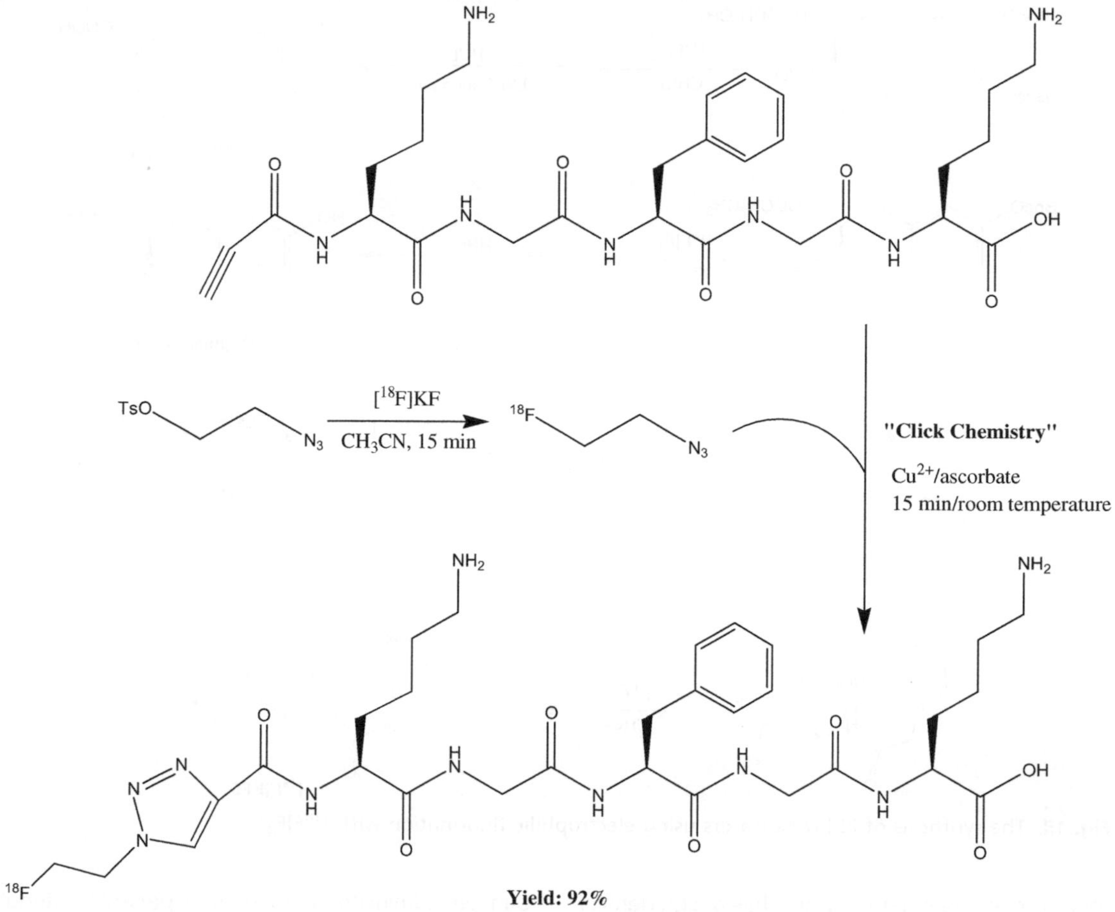

Fig. 12. Click chemistry and an example of its use in ^{18}F-labeled peptide chemistry. (*Data from* Glaser M and E Arstad. "Click labeling" with 2-[^{18}F]fluoroethylazide for positron emission tomography. Bioconjug Chem 2007;18(3):989–93.)

radiotracer for ligand binding site on the protein, and the level of nonspecific binding of the tracer. Tracers having a high affinity (ie picomolar) for the target receptor often bind irreversibly to the receptor. That is, there is no washout of radiotracer from regions of the brain expressing the receptor during the data acquisition period of PET. The uptake of tracers displaying irreversible kinetics in vivo can be dependent on and influenced by differences in cerebral blood flow. Therefore, kinetically irreversible tracers often require correction for differences in cerebral blood flow (ie, [^{15}O]water study or K_1 estimates by analyzing the early part of the tissue-time activity curves) to obtain accurate measures of the density or binding potential of the receptor or protein under investigation. A prime example of this concept is the development of PET radiotracers for imaging striatal versus extrastriatal D_2/D_3 receptors. [^{11}C]Raclopride, which has ~5 nM affinity for D_2 and D_3 receptors, is a suitable radiotracer for imaging striatal D_2/D_3 receptors. There is a high density of D_2/D_3 receptors in the caudate and putamen and the tracer binds reversibly to D_2/D_3 receptors. However, it is not generally useful for imaging extrastriatal D_2/D_3 receptors, which are expressed in lower density in dopamine receptor–enriched extrastriatal regions versus the caudate and putamen. The short half-life of ^{11}C and rapid dissociation of [^{11}C]raclopride from dopamine receptors results in a low signal-to-noise ratio in regions with a low density of D_2/D_3 receptors. The best radiotracers for imaging extrastriatal D_2/D_3 receptors are [^{18}F]fallypride and [^{18}F]FLB-457, which have a picomolar affinity for D_2 and D_3 receptors, and a low level of nonspecific binding. These properties (picomolar affinity and low nonspecific binding) make it possible to obtain stable measures of extrastriatal receptors expressing in brain regions containing a low density of D_2 and D_3 receptors. The irreversible binding of [^{18}F]fallypride and [^{18}F]FLB-457 to D_2/D_3

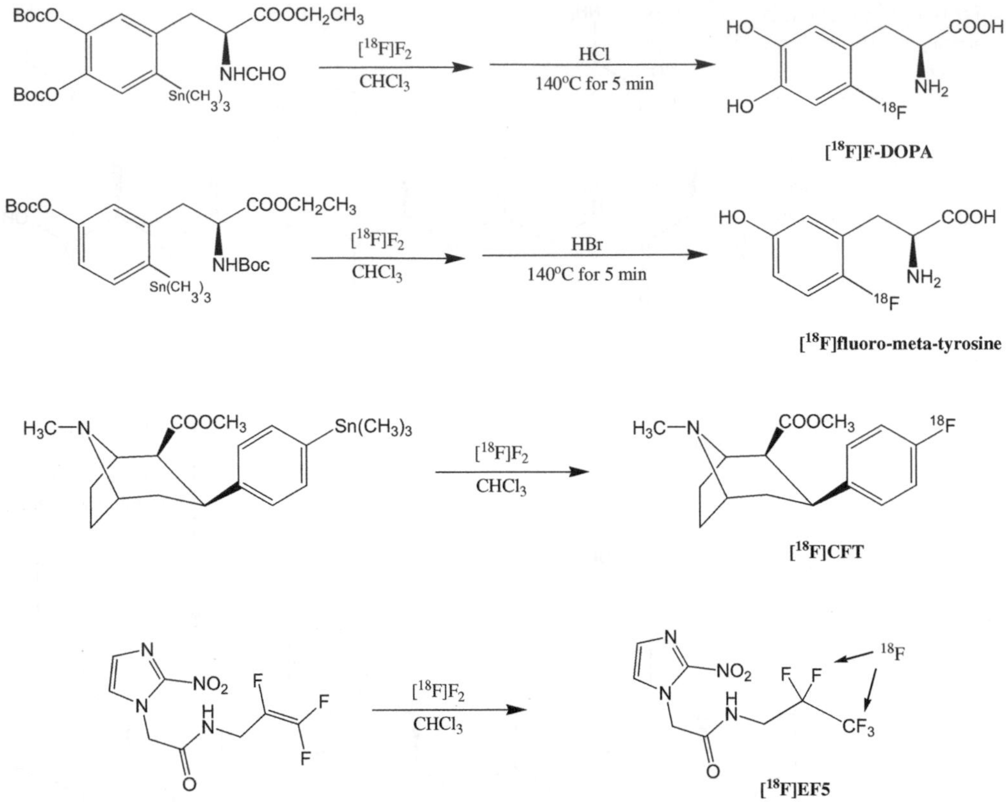

Fig. 13. The synthesis of PET radiotracers using electrophilic fluorination with $[^{18}F]F_2$.

receptors in the striatum, which has a high density of D_2 and D_3 receptors, requires a correction for differences in cerebral blood flow to obtain an accurate measure of the D_2/D_3 receptor binding potential.

Specific Activity

Specific activity is also a factor that must be considered for PET imaging studies in which there is a saturable level of receptor or target protein. The lower the target density (eg, B_{max}), the higher the specific activity needed to ensure that the principles of radiotracer binding are maintained (ie, only a small percentage of sites are occupied by the radioligands). Because specific activity changes with time, the more useful measurement in PET radiotracer formulations is the amount of mass contained in the dose. For ^{11}C- and ^{18}F-labeled radiotracers, 1 to 10 μg of cold compound are usually synthesized because of the presence of carrier in the target materials and reagents. The amount of mass that can be injected in the patient depends on the density of the target being imaged, as well as the pharmacology or toxicology of the compound. Typically 0.5 to 5 μg of carrier can be administered to human patients without any adverse side-effects.

Lipophilicity and Other Physicochemical Properties

Because most CNS-based radiotracers cross the blood-brain barrier by a passive diffusion mechanism, the main physicochemical property of a PET radiotracer that determines its ability to enter the brain and label the target receptor or enzyme is the lipophilicity of the compound. Lipophilicity is operationally defined as the logarithm of the octanol-water partition coefficient of the compound (ie, the logP value). There is a parabolic relationship between the brain uptake and the logP of a PET radiotracer. The optimal range of logP values for a CNS radiotracer is 2.0 to 3.5, but radiotracers with logP values higher than 4.0 are also capable of crossing the blood-brain barrier, albeit at a lower value. Increasing the logP value also results in a higher amount of nonspecific binding of the radiotracer, which can be problematic for imaging targets with a low expression in the brain. Other factors that can influence the ability of a compound to cross the blood-brain barrier by a passive diffusion mechanism are the molecular weight and number of hydrogen donors or acceptors in the molecule. Compounds with a molecular weight greater than 600 g/mol or less than 6 H bonds have a lower tendency to cross the blood-brain barrier. In addition, radiotracers displaying a high level of protein binding have a low free fraction and typically do not show high uptake in brain.

Metabolism

Because PET measures only the radioactive decay of a positron emitter, one must confirm that a PET radiotracer for imaging targets within the CNS does not undergo peripheral metabolism in a manner that results in the formation of radiolabeled metabolites capable of crossing the blood-brain barrier. The formation of lipophilic radiolabeled metabolites complicates the use of graphical or compartmental methods of radiotracer modeling because one must know the level of signal in the brain caused by the metabolite in addition to the parent compound, which is technically challenging. Consequently, most radiotracers used in quantitative imaging studies of CNS targets are metabolized in a manner that does not lead to the formation of lipophilic radiolabeled metabolites capable of crossing the blood-brain barrier. The metabolism rate of the radiolabeled compound can also affect the brain uptake of a radiotracer. Radiotracers that are rapidly metabolized (completely between 5 and 10 minutes after injection) typically have a low brain uptake because PET radiotracers usually reach peak uptake in brain between 10 and 30 minutes after injection.

FACTORS USED IN THE DESIGN OF PET RADIOTRACERS

One of the advantages of $[^{11}C]CH_3I$ and $[^{11}C]CH_3OTf$ in the development of PET radiotracers is that there are many lead compounds in the literature that have an *N*-methyl group in the parent structure that simplifies the development of an ^{11}C-labeled radiotracer. In this case, an ^{11}C-labeled radiotracer can be prepared by reacting the corresponding *des*-methyl precursor with $[^{11}C]CH_3I/[^{11}C]CH_3OTf$. Consequently, the ^{11}C-labeled analogue is a true radiotracer because the ^{11}C is incorporated in the parent compound. This situation is occasionally true with ^{18}F-labeled radiotracers, and $[^{18}F]$setoperone and $[^{18}F]$NMSP are examples where an ^{18}F for ^{19}F substitution leads to a straightforward preparation of an ^{18}F-labed radiotracer. However, in many cases this is not an option, and an ^{11}C- or ^{18}F-labeled radiotracer must be designed using a lead compound whose structure must be altered in a way to incorporate the ^{11}C or ^{18}F radiolabel. In this case, the radiolabel must be introduced into the lead compound in a manner that does not reduce the affinity of the ligand for the target macromolecule. Some of the logic used by radiochemists in the design of PET radiotracers using a lead compound in which there is no simple method (ie, hot-for-cold atom substitution) for accomplishing this goal is discussed later.

Table 2 provides several substituents used to design PET radiotracers in which the structure of the lead compound must be altered to incorporate a positron-emitting radionuclide. The left-hand column of **Table 2** shows the primary radionuclides and common labeling strategies for incorporating ^{11}C or ^{18}F into a lead compound. The second column shows the Hansch lipophilicity constant (π) value for each substituent; the π value is a measure of the relative lipophilicity of the substituent and determines the effect of adding this substituent on the overall logP of the molecule.[63] For example, replacing an H atom of a lead compound with a methyl group will increase the logP value by 0.56 units. The third column lists the Hammet substituent constant (σ_p), which is a measure of the electron-withdrawing or electron-donating properties of the substituent. A negative σ_p value indicates the substituent donates electrons to an aromatic ring system, whereas a positive σ_p constant indicates that this is an electron-withdrawing substituent. The molar refractivity (MR) of the substituent is a measure of the steric bulk of each functional group.

Substitution of an H atom of a primary or secondary amine with an $[^{11}C]$methyl group is

Table 2
Substituent constants for radionuclides and labeling strategies used in PET radiotracer development

Substituent	π	σ_p	MR
H	0.00	0.00	0.1
OH	−0.67	−0.37	2.85
CH_3	0.56	−0.17	0.57
F	0.14	0.06	0.1
I	1.12	0.18	1.39
Br	0.86	0.23	0.89
CH_2CH_2F	0.85	−0.15	0.93
$CH_2CH_2CH_2F$	1.59	–	1.48

Data from Hansch C, Leo A, Hoekman D. Exploring QSAR: hydrophobic, electronic, and steric constants. In: Heller SR, editor. Computer applications in chemistry, vol. 2. Washington, DC: American Chemical Society; 1995. p. 348.

a commonly used strategy provided that there is enough steric tolerance in the region of the nitrogen atom (MR for a CH_3 group = 0.57 vs 0.1 for an H atom). Substitution of a CH_3 for an H atom also increases the lipophilicity of the PET radiotracer by 0.56 π units, which results in a higher degree of nonspecific binding relative to the parent compound.

The synthesis of ^{18}F-labeled compounds often involves the substitution of an F for H, which rarely alters the affinity and physicochemical properties of the parent compound because the substituent constants of an F atom are similar to those of an H atom. However, F is also capable of serving as a hydrogen bond acceptor; therefore, a second case that has been used in the design of ^{18}F-labeled radiotracers is a substitution of an F atom for an OH group.

The use of a 2-fluoroethyl or 3-fluoropropyl group for introducing ^{18}F into a lead compound is increasing in popularity because the radiochemical yields of an SN2 reaction are generally high. However, the substituent constants in terms of lipophilicity (π) and steric bulk (MR) limits the options in which these groups can be substituted into a lead compound. For example, the substitution of a 2-fluoroethyl or 3-fluoropropyl group for an H atom is not optimal because it would result in a large increase in the lipophilicity (ie, logP) of the compound, and also introduces a quantity of steric bulk into the region of the molecule in which the substitution occurs. A 2-fluoroethyl or 3-fluoropropyl for methyl substitution can work provided that (1) the increase in lipophilicity does not increase the nonspecific binding to the point that the tracer does not have a suitable signal-to-noise ratio for imaging purposes, and (2) the increased steric bulk does not reduce the affinity of the ligand for the target protein. A more appropriate substitution is a 2-fluoroethyl group for a Br atom, and a 3-fluoropropyl group for an I atom. Note the similarity in the substituent constants for the 2-fluoroethyl group and a Br atom, and the 3-fluoropropyl group for an I atom. In addition, because many CNS-active compounds contain either a Br or I atom in the parent structure, this strategy often leads to the development of a successful PET radiotracer without the need to conduct a rigorous structure-activity relationship study. Examples of the different strategies for PET radiotracer design are shown in **Fig. 14**.

PRECLINICAL EVALUATION OF NEW RADIOTRACERS

The initial evaluation of a PET radiotracer for imaging receptors or proteins within the CNS typically involves studies in rodents (usually rats) aimed at determining whether the radiotracer crosses the blood-brain barrier and labels the target protein in vivo. For receptor-based radiotracers, blocking studies are usually performed with a gold standard blocking agent to determine the specificity of the radiotracer for the target receptor. Because the metabolism of radiotracers in rodents is different from that of humans, ex vivo metabolism studies in rodents are typically not performed because the data may not be predictive of what occurs in primates. The poor performance of a PET radiotracer in rodents does not guarantee a similar poor performance in higher species such as nonhuman primates, largely because of species differences in metabolism; it is the authors' standard practice to conduct at least 1 imaging study in nonhuman primates before eliminating a radiotracer from further investigation.

The best animal model for evaluating new PET radiotracers for imaging CNS function is macaque monkeys (ie, rhesus or cynomolgus monkeys). Because macaque monkeys are phylogenetically closer to humans than rodents, radiotracers that produce promising PET imaging results in monkeys typically succeed in clinical research studies in humans. These preclinical studies include a battery of tests such as evaluating the between-subject and test/retest variability of the radiotracer, blood metabolism, and in vivo blocking or displacement studies to confirm specificity of the radiotracer for its molecular target.

A unique feature of conducting PET imaging studies in macaque monkeys is that there are several nonhuman primate models of behavior and disease that are predictive of, and often parallel, different neurologic and behavioral conditions in humans. Examples of these models include the 1-methyl-4-phenyl-1,2,3,6-tetrahydropyridine (MPTP) model of Parkinson disease,[64,65] cocaine self-administration,[3,4] nonhuman primate models of socially derived stress,[66,67] and age-related cognitive impairment.[68] These animal models not only serve as a screening tool for evaluating new radiotracers for subsequent clinical research studies but also provide a unique resource for designing PET imaging studies capable of addressing specific neurobiological questions that cannot be conducted in human imaging studies. An example of this was the study by Nader and colleagues,[67] in which a rhesus monkey model of cocaine self-administration was used to assess the effect of acute and chronic exposure to cocaine on dopamine receptor function in cocaine-naive animals.

Once a PET radiotracer has shown promising results in preclinical PET imaging studies

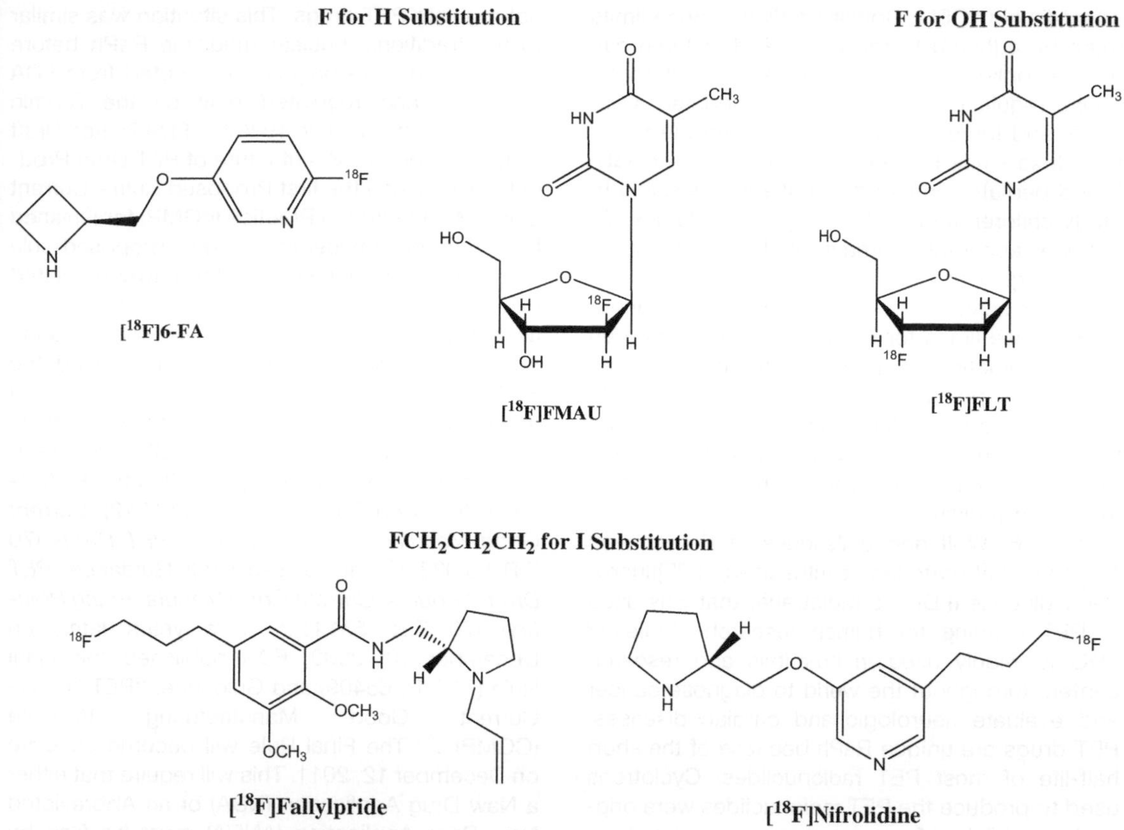

Fig. 14. Examples of ^{18}F radiotracer development.

conducted in nonhuman primates, then a series of steps must be taken before its use in human subjects. Unlike animal research, which is governed by the Department of Agriculture and the American Association for Laboratory Animal Care, PET imaging studies in humans are under the regulatory control of the US Food and Drug Administration (FDA). A brief description of the regulatory criteria for producing PET radiotracers for clinical imaging studies is presented in the next section.

REGULATION OF PET RADIOTRACER PRODUCTION FOR USE IN HUMANS: HISTORICAL PERSPECTIVE AND CURRENT STATUS

From 1963 to 1975 the FDA exempted all radioactive drugs from compliance with new drug requirements, as long as they complied with the Atomic Energy Commission regulations. In 1975 the FDA lifted this exemption, and together with the newly formed Nuclear Regulatory Commission, required that all radioactive drug manufacturers be subject to the requirements of the Food Drug and Cosmetic Act (FD&C Act). The FDA also required that all human research studies involving radiopharmaceuticals (RaPh) be carried out under an investigational new drug (IND) application. In addition, in 1975, the Radioactive Drug Research Committee (RDRC) regulations were established in Title 21 Code of Federal Regulations part 361.1; these regulations clarified under what situations certain radioactive drugs would be eligible for use in basic research studies involving human subjects, without requiring an IND. To establish an RDRC at an Academic Institution, members are appointed by the Institution. The committee is composed of physicians and scientists who are required to cover specific specialty areas. Each RDRC is approved by the FDA and must report at least annually regarding its activities.

The RDRC permits basic research in humans, but does not allow first-in-human studies. In addition, no clinical decisions are allowed under RDRC regulated research. The pharmacology of the drug must be known in humans and generally recognized as safe and effective. No observed pharmacologic effects can be noted from the mass dose administered. This is referred to at the no observed effect level (NOEL). Specific radiation dose limits must be adhered to for adults, and children can receive only 10% of the allowable adult limits. These regulations have not been updated since 1975, and there are problems meeting the radiation dose limits for pediatric studies. The established pediatric limits often make it impossible to study children under RDRC regulated studies. To acquire acceptable image statistics, pediatric PET imaging studies can require administration of higher dosages than would be allowed under RDRC dose limits for children. This situation can be problematic for grant funding that requires inclusion of pediatric subjects in the research. In such instances, an IND must then be filed with the FDA to proceed with pediatric studies. **Fig. 15** shows the regulatory process, modified from VanBrocklin.[69]

In 1976, Wolf and colleagues at Brookhaven National Laboratories synthesized [^{18}F]fluorodeoxyglucose (FDG), a radiotracer that was used in PET imaging for human research studies.[70] FDG is widely used in hospitals and research centers throughout the world to diagnose cancer and evaluate neurologic and cardiac diseases. PET drugs are unique RaPh because of the short half-life of most PET radionuclides. Cyclotrons used to produce the PET radionuclides were originally established for research purposes in university settings. Each batch of a PET drug was prepared and administered for research purposes only on the day of preparation for a single patient injection. Regulation of these research studies usually proceeded under the RDRC or through IND submission at respective universities. During the 1980s and 1990s, interest in FDG for possible clinical use increased. During this time the FDA did not regulate PET drugs. This situation was similar to the traditional nuclear medicine RaPh before 1975, which were originally exempted from FDA oversight, and regulated only by the Atomic Energy Commission. In 1995 the FDA issued Draft Guidelines on the Manufacture of PET Drug Products, and issued the first Proposed Rule—Current Good Manufacturing Practice (cGMP) for Finished PET Radiopharmaceuticals. This proposed rule met significant concern from the newly regulated PET community, and congress was mobilized by its constituency. By 1997 the FDA Modernization Act (FDAMA) was finalized, which required the FDA to develop appropriate current good manufacturing practice standards for PET drugs, which would be separate from cGMP for traditional drugs. On September 20, 2005 the FDA issued Proposed Rule (21 CFR Part §212): *Current Good Manufacturing Practice for PET Drugs* (70 F.R 55,038),[71] and revised Draft Guidance: *PET Drug Products: Current Good Manufacturing Practice* (70 F.R. 55145).[72] Five years later, on December 10, 2009, FDA published the Final Rule (74 F.R. 65409) and Guidance, "PET Drugs–Current Good Manufacturing Practice (CGMP)".[73] The Final Rule will become effective on December 12, 2011. This will require that either a New Drug Application (NDA) or an Abbreviated New Drug Application (ANDA) must be filed by each manufacturer, before the effective date, for the existing FDA approved PET drugs, F-18 fluorodeoxyglucose, F-18 fluoride, and N-13 ammonia.

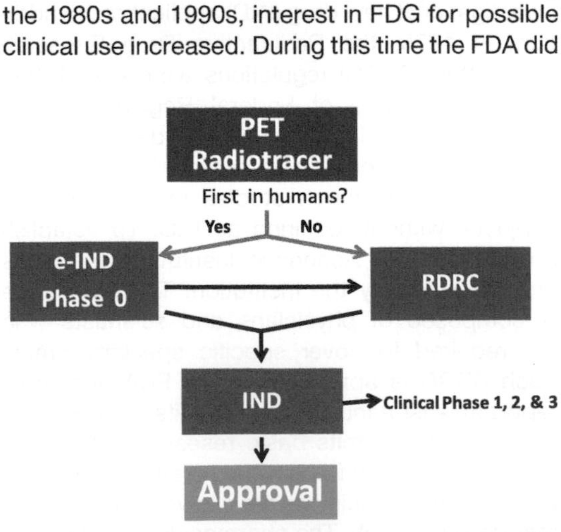

Fig. 15. FDA regulatory process for new PET radiotracers. (*Data from* VanBrocklin HF. Radiopharmaceuticals for drug development: United States regulatory perspective. Current radiopharmaceuticals 2008;1(1):2–6.)

Until the effective date, PET drug compounding (manufacturing) remains subject to the provisions of Section 121 of FDAMA, requiring that the compounding (manufacturing) of PET drugs must conform to the requirements of the United States Phamacopeia (USP) Chapter 823 *Radiopharmaceuticals for Positron Emission Tomography—Compounding*,[74] and if available, USP monographs. The Final Rule, will allow a PET drug producer to follow 21 CFR Part 212 or continue to use USP chapter 823 for the production of investigational PET drugs produced under an IND (phase 1 and 2) and research drugs produced under the authority of the RDRC. If a PET drug producer intends to seek marketing approval for a PET drug, phase 3 studies of the drug should be in accordance with the PET CGMP requirements in 21 CFR Part 212.

THE EXPLORATORY IND MECHANISM AND ITS EFFECT ON FIRST-IN-HUMAN STUDIES

Because PET RPh are true tracers, they contain a minimal mass quantity and have no expected pharmacologic or toxicologic effects. Yet in the past they were required to provide the same safety evaluation as traditional drugs. This process required significant monetary resources; the cost of the pharmacologic and toxicology studies alone for a traditional IND ranged between US$400,000 and US$500,000.[69]

Because of the significant decline during the past 15 years in numbers of submissions to the FDA for new molecular entities and biologics, the FDA developed a plan called the Critical Path Initiative, which served as a framework for facilitating drug discovery and development.[75] One of the initiatives the FDA implemented in 2006 was to develop guidance describing the flexibility that existed in the IND program to allow testing of multiple candidate drugs in the early clinical phases.[76] For PET drug development, this has significantly affected imaging probe development. The Exploratory Investigational New Drug (eIND) embraces the concept of microdosing, which was initially introduced in the European Union in 2004 by a position paper.[77] The microdose mass is one-hundredth of the dose of a test substance calculated to yield a pharmacologic effect. The maximum allowable mass dose is 100 μg or less, or for protein products 30 nmoles or less. If the mass requirement is met, there are reduced pharmacology and toxicology requirements. This system also significantly reduces the cost to bring a new drug to market. For the eIND toxicology study only 1 mammalian species is required, and both sexes must be studied. The administered mass dose must be at least 100 times the anticipated mass dose to be administered in the human. The length of the toxicology study must be 14 days, with interim necropsy on day 2 and on day 14. A limited subject enrollment of 5 to 30 subjects is allowed. Under the eIND only the phase 0 studies are performed, and if the candidate drug is successful, and further study is indicated, a transition to the traditional IND phase 1 must be completed. This limited IND facilitates first-in-human imaging studies for drugs and biologics, and bridges the gap between the preclinical and clinical trials. It is ideal for proof-of-concept studies, and testing of multiple candidate drugs to identify a lead candidate to move forward through the IND process. As molecular imaging advances, these changes in the regulatory environment should stimulate the development of RaPh in a more cost-effective manner.

USP CHAPTER 823 QUALITY CONTROL REQUIREMENTS FOR PET RAPH

PET drug production involves use of short-lived cyclotron-produced radionuclides, which are then incorporated into the final drug product. These radiolabeled drugs require significant considerations because of the half-lives (which vary from minutes to hours) and decay emissions (positrons and 511 keV photons) requiring significant radioprotection. In addition the short half-lives necessitate rapid quality control methods, to assure the batch is acceptable for intravenous injection in humans. Because sterility testing requires 14 days to complete, the product must be released before the completion of sterility testing. This system requires additional aseptic process controls are in place to ensure the quality of the final product.

As mentioned earlier, PET drugs must be compounded (manufactured) according to USP Chapter 823. This regulation requires that written specifications must be in place for the identity, purity, and quality of all components used for any PET drug compounding procedure, which includes definition of the appropriate storage. All shipments of components must follow a log-in process and expiration dates must be recorded. If there is no expiration date, one must be assigned. For acceptance of a lot of sterile filters, a sample filter must be tested for integrity. Manufacturers' certificates of analysis can be used to demonstrate compliance with the established written specifications.

Chapter 823 also requires written acceptance criteria be established for each PET drug defining the identity, purity, and quality of the finished PET drug. If a USP monograph exists, these standards are the minimum acceptance criteria. Written and verified procedures must be established for each PET drug that incorporates 0.22 μm sterile membrane filtration for parenteral administration or 0.45 μm particulate filtration for PET drugs intended for inhalation.

Controls must be maintained of computers and related automated equipment to ensure that changes in compounding software are instituted by authorized personnel. It is also required to document and verify changes and assure that only the current version of the software is being used in PET compounding. Copies of outdated software must be kept to provide a complete history from the time of initiation of a synthesis.

Verification studies must be performed on a minimum of 3 consecutive batches of a new PET drug to show that the product meets established acceptance criteria. In addition, whenever there is a change in the compounding procedure, computer software program, or component specifications that have the potential to alter the identity, quality, or purity of the drug product, 3 consecutive verification studies must again be performed.

Expiration dating and storage conditions for the PET drug must be established on the results of stability testing. The test samples must be withdrawn from the product stored in the container used for the PET drug. The PET drug must meet all acceptance criteria at expiration.

Before initiating the PET synthesis, the sterile filter and vent filters must be inserted through the final PET product vial septum in a class 100 environment (laminar flow hood or isolator). The internal surfaces of the class 100 hood must be disinfected with a sterile disinfectant such as 70% isopropyl alcohol before use. Microbiological testing should be performed periodically using microbiological contact plates for the surfaces and settle plates or a dynamic air sampler.

The PET drug must be compounded according to a written verified standard operating procedure, and a batch record must be maintained for each batch of drug produced. Lot numbers of the PET drug must initial all the critical steps, indicating that they were performed. Any unplanned deviation or unexpected results must be documented and investigated. This documentation should be in writing. All analytical data must be included with each batch record.

For PET drugs with a half-life of 20 minutes or greater the following quality control testing requirements must be completed on the batch, or for PET drugs with a half-life of 20 minutes or less the quality control should be performed on the initial subbatch, before release, according to established written procedures. The quality control subbatch is the first batch of a PET drug made from a single lot of components, for example [^{15}O]water or [^{13}N]ammonia. The following are the test procedures required.

1. For all PET drugs intended for parenteral administration a membrane filter integrity test must be completed after final filtration. The bubble point test is commonly performed, which requires use of a pressure gauge and a source of air pressure connected to the transfer set attached to the filter used for the synthesis. The pressure is increased until the validated bubble point is reached. This test must be completed before release for human use, except in the case of [^{15}O]water, in which the integrity test may be completed after injection.
2. The pH must be measured, usually using pH paper.
3. The PET drug must be visually inspected using adequate shielding for an as-low-as-reasonably-achievable technique, to ensure the solution that is clear and free of particulate matter.
4. Radiochemical purity and identity are analyzed using thin-layer or high-pressure liquid radiochromatography. A nonradioactive standard must be chromatographed with the PET drug to allow identification of the compound, using an authentic standard for comparison with the radiolabeled drug. If a USP standard is available, it must be used. The FDA, cGMP for PET (21 CFR Part §212.70) Final Rule states that conditional final release cannot be granted if tests for radiochemical purity and identity are not performed. Radiochemical purity analysis may require duplication of quality control equipment.
5. Radionuclidic identity: identity testing involves decay analysis in a dose calibrator for a defined period. The half-life is determined mathematically using linear regression.
6. Specific activity analysis is required for PET drugs with mass-dependent localization or toxicity concerns. An example of a PET drug requiring specific activity analysis is a radiotracer for imaging receptor function such as [^{11}C]raclopride.
7. Residual solvent analysis and other toxic chemicals (such as Kryptofix-222) must be analyzed to determine compliance with established acceptance criteria. Gas chromatographic methods can be developed for the measurement of residual solvents that allow precision and linearity across the range of concentration levels required by the USP Chapter 467.[78] There is a USP-approved method for Kryptofix analysis in the FDG monograph. In addition there are other methods, such as the Mock method,[79] using iodoplatinate thin-layer chromatography strips to perform a color end-point test, which can be validated for Kryptofix analysis.[78]
8. Bacterial endotoxin testing (BET) must be performed. A 60-minute bacterial endotoxin test (gel-clot) or other recognized test such as the photometric test must be performed on each batch. The acceptable endotoxin limit is 175 endotoxin units/V. The V is usually defined as the batch volume of the PET drug.

Postrelease sterility testing must be performed for each batch of PET drug. The USP 823 currently requires that the product must be inoculated in fluid thioglycolate and soybean-casein digest media within 24 hours after the end of synthesis. The PET cGMP Final Rule has increased this time to 30 hours. If the microbiological test fails, an investigation needs to be performed to determine the cause, and the corrective actions that will be taken. It is good to maintain all these records in writing to assure an adequate record. After a record of successful sterility tests is established for a particular PET drug, only the first lot prepared each day needs to be subjected to a sterility test, unless the second batch of that PET drug uses any components that differ from the first batch.

The USP monographs require that radionuclidic purity should be determined, but do not specify the time interval. γ-Ray spectroscopy using a suitable γ counting device such as a multichannel analyzer can be used to determine the presence of any γ photon energy other than that characteristic of positron-emitting radionuclides, which would include 511 keV, 1.02 MeV, or Compton scatter.

All aseptic operations used in producing PET drugs, including assembly of sterile components, compounding, filtration, and manipulation of sterile solutions, must be performed by operators, qualified to work with aseptic techniques. Operators must be qualified by passing three growth promotion tests, which require process simulations using microbiological growth medium. After simulation, the media are incubated at the appropriate temperature for 14 days with periodic examination for the evidence of bacterial growth. The absence of growth is necessary for an acceptable test result. Simulations are performed in triplicate to qualify a new operator. After initial qualification, 1 simulation must be performed each year, or each time procedures are changed. All aseptic operations are performed by operators wearing appropriate laboratory clothing.

USP CHAPTER 797 OVERVIEW

In the case of production of RaPh for PET, USP Chapter 823 supersedes Chapter 797 *Pharmaceutical Compounding–Sterile Preparations*.[80] On release of a PET drug as a finished drug product from a production facility, the further handling, manipulation, or use of the product is considered compounding, and the contents of Chapter 797 are applicable. Chapter 797 sets out practice standards to help ensure that compounded sterile preparations (CSPs) are of high quality. These standards help to ensure that these compounded products do not inflict harm on patients as a result of contaminated preparations, and assigns risk levels according to potential for microbial contamination during compounding. Although PET production is not required to follow Chapter 797, it outlines practices required for PET drug dispensing, and a general overview of the chapter is discussed in the following section.

One of the sections of Chapter 797 is Radiopharmaceuticals As CSPs. This section describes RaPh, compounded from sterile components in closed sterile containers, with a volume of 100 mL or less, and a single-dose injection of not more than 30 mL, as low-risk level CSPs. Low-risk CSPs must have a 12-hour or less expiration time or beyond-use time.

Low-risk RaPh are compounded from sterile components in an International Organization for Standardization (ISO) class 5 (enclosures allow 100 particles of 0.5 μm and larger per cubic foot of air) primary engineering control (PEC) with not more than 2 entries into the original sterile vial. The ISO class 5 PEC must be located in an ISO class 8 (enclosures allow 100,000 particles of 0.5 μm and larger per cubic foot of air) area or a segregated compounding area. The area may be demarcated by a line on the floor, or be a separate room. The room must have no unsealed windows, and no connection to outside, or areas of high traffic flow. There must be no sink next to the ISO class 5 PEC. Personnel must be appropriately gowned and gloved in the work area.

Immediate-use provision is intended only for those situations when there is a need for emergency or immediate patient administration of a CSP. Immediate-use CSPs are exempt from low-risk RaPh requirements if the RaPh can be prepared, dispensed, and administered within 1 hour of preparation. An example of an immediate-use practice in PET would be the dispensing of an ^{11}C-labeled PET RaPh, prepared for a single patient administration.

Chapter 797 outlines aseptic training requirements to compound low-risk RaPh, and they can be used as guidance for setting up training for preparation of PET drugs. Training can be achieved using audiovisual instruction sources, produced by expert personnel, as well as written publications. Personnel are required to pass a written examination after training, and initially complete media-fill testing, using aseptic manipulations, to demonstrate compounding skills. This testing must be repeated at least annually. This training differs from the Chapter 823 requirements for completion of 3 media-fill tests before being initially authorized to compound PET drugs.

Written training procedures are required for appropriate gowning and gloving, including procedures for hand washing. Gowning requirements include dedicated shoes or shoe covers, head cover, masks and eye protection, gowns with fitted sleeves, and sterile gloves disinfected with sterile 70% isopropanol. These training procedures must be documented through observational audits and gloved fingertip sampling using microbiological contact plates. Garb exposed in patient care areas may not reenter the compounding area.

USP Chapter 797 requires the ISO class 5 PEC must be cleaned using appropriate disinfectants (such as 70% sterile isopropyl alcohol alternated on a defined schedule with a disinfectant effective against spore-forming bacteria) at the beginning of each shift, and checked regularly using contact and air-settling plates. The value of viable microbial monitoring of gloved fingertips and surfaces of components and the compounding environment is to identify and correct unacceptable work practice. Chapter 797 recommended action levels for microbial contamination are in an ISO class 5 environment, fingertip samples should be greater than 3 colony-forming units (cfu) per plate and surface sample testing (contact plate) should also be greater than 3 cfu per plate. For ISO class 8 surface sampling action levels should be greater than 100 cfu per plate. If these levels are exceeded work practices and cleaning procedures should be reevaluated. An investigation should be initiated until the source of the problem is eliminated, the area is cleaned (or task), and resampling is successfully performed. This investigation may require review of hand hygiene, garbing, and gloving.

Because most PET drugs are administered intravenously, it is important to emphasize the aseptic process without placing undue burden on that process with additional regulatory requirements. All PET drug batches are released after most quality control requirements are completed. Although sterility testing is not complete the final filter is tested for integrity and the BET test is completed, giving an indication of the sterility of the final PET drug. The mass of drug contained in a PET drug is usually in the μg range, compared with therapeutic drugs, which allows an additional safety factor for PET drugs.

SUMMARY

The development of ^{11}C- and ^{18}F-labeled probes for use with PET continues to be an active area of research. ^{11}C will continue to be a useful radiotracer in clinical research studies because the short half-life of this radionuclide (20.4 minutes) permits imaging sessions in which multiple tracers can be administered (following a short delay to allow for radioactive decay and biologic clearance). Therefore, 2 or more targets comprising a biochemical pathway or neurotransmitter system can be studied in the same imaging session when using ^{11}C-labeled radiotracers. ^{18}F will continue to be the radionuclide of choice for imaging studies using a single radiotracer. Advances in ^{18}F-labeling strategies such as the development of click chemistry will likely have an effect on the future development of ^{18}F-labeled radiotracers. Recent changes in the regulatory requirements such as the creation of the eIND and phase 0 studies in humans are expected to lead to a dramatic increase in the number of PET radiotracers making the translational jump from preclinical research studies in animal models of disease to clinical research studies in patients. However, the continued success in translational PET research studies using new PET radiotracers depends on the strict adherence of PET radiochemistry programs to the requirements stated in the USP Chapter 823 *Radiopharmaceuticals for Positron Emission Tomography—Compounding*, or the new 35 CFR Part 212.

ACKNOWLEDGMENTS

The authors would like to thank Lynne Jones for her excellent editorial assistance.

REFERENCES

1. Luedtke RR, Mach RH. Progress in developing D3 dopamine receptor ligands as potential therapeutic agents for neurological and neuropsychiatric disorders. Curr Pharm Des 2003;9(8):643–71.
2. Ryoo HL, Pierrotti D, Joyce JN. Dopamine D3 receptor is decreased and D2 receptor is elevated in the striatum of Parkinson's disease. Mov Disord 1998;13(5):788–97.
3. Moore RJ, et al. Effect of cocaine self-administration on dopamine D2 receptors in rhesus monkeys. Synapse 1998;30(1):88–96.
4. Nader MA, et al. PET imaging of dopamine D2 receptors during chronic cocaine self-administration in monkeys. Nat Neurosci 2006;9(8):1050–6.
5. Volkow ND, Fowler JS, Wang GJ, et al. Dopamine in drug abuse and addiction: results from imaging studies and treatment implications. Mol Psychiatry 2004;9(6):557–69.
6. Volkow ND, Fowler JS, Wolf AP, et al. Effects of chronic cocaine abuse on postsynaptic dopamine receptors. Am J Psychiatry 1990;147(6):719–24.
7. Staley JK, Mash DC. Adaptive increase in D3 dopamine receptors in the brain reward circuits of human cocaine fatalities. J Neurosci 1996;16(19):6100–6.
8. Hannon J, Hoyer D. Molecular biology of 5-HT receptors. Behav Brain Res 2008;195(1):198–213.
9. Carroll FI. Antagonists at metabotropic glutamate receptor subtype 5: structure activity relationships and therapeutic potential for addiction. Ann N Y Acad Sci 2008;1141:221–32.
10. Hein L. Adrenoceptors and signal transduction in neurons. Cell Tissue Res 2006;326(2):541–51.
11. Harper DB, O'Hagan D. The fluorinated natural products. Nat Prod Rep 1994;11(2):123–33.

12. Filler R, Kobayashi Y, Yagulpolskii LM. Organofluorine compounds in medicinal chemistry and biomedical applications. Studies in Organic Chemistry, vol. 48. Amsterdam (The Netherlands): Elsevier; 1993. p. 394.
13. Hammadi A, Crouzel C. Synthesis of [18F]-(S)-fluoxetine: a selective serotonine uptake inhibitor. J Labelled Comp Radiopharm 1993;33(8):703–10.
14. Das MK, Mukherjee J. Radiosynthesis of [F-18]fluoxetine as a potential radiotracer for serotonin reuptake sites. Appl Radiat Isot 1993;44(5):835–42.
15. Suehiro M, Wilson AA, Scheffel U, et al. Radiosynthesis and evaluation of N-(3-[18F]fluoropropyl)paroxetine as a radiotracer for in vivo labeling of serotonin uptake sites by PET. Nucl Med Biol 1991; 18(7):791–6.
16. Shiue CY, Fowler JS, Wolf AP, et al. Syntheses and specific activity determinations of no-carrier-added (NCA) F-18-labeled butyrophenone neuroleptics–benperidol, haloperidol, spiroperidol, and pipamperone. J Nucl Med 1985;26(2):181–6.
17. Hamacher K, Hamkens W. Remote controlled one-step production of 18F labeled butyrophenone neuroleptics exemplified by the synthesis of n.c.a. [18F] N-methylspiperone. Appl Radiat Isot 1995;46(9): 911–6.
18. Katsifis A, Hamacher K, Schnitter J, et al. Optimization studies concerning the direct nucleophilic fluorination of butyrophenone neuroleptics. Appl Radiat Isot 1993;44(7):1015–20.
19. Crouzel C, Venet M, Irie T, et al. Labeling of a serotoninergic ligand with 18F: [18F] setoperone. J Labelled Comp Radiopharm 1988;25(4): 403–14.
20. Mach RH, Luedtke RR, Unsworth CD, et al. 18F-labeled benzamides for studying the dopamine D2 receptor with positron emission tomography. J Med Chem 1993;36(23):3707–20.
21. Schlyer DJ. PET tracers and radiochemistry. Ann Acad Med Singapore 2004;33(2):146–54.
22. Elsinga PH. Radiopharmaceutical chemistry for positron emission tomography. Methods 2002; 27(3):208–17.
23. Pike V, Eakins M, Allan R, et al. Preparation of carbon-11 labelled acetate and palmitic acid for the study of myocardial metabolism by emission-computerised axial tomography. J Radioanal Nucl Chem 1981;64(1):291–7.
24. McCarron JA, Turton DR, Pike VW, et al. Remotely-controlled production of the 5-HT1A receptor radioligand, [carbonyl-11C]WAY-100635, via 11C-carboxylation of an immobilized Grignard reagent. J Labelled Comp Radiopharm 1996; 38(10):941–53.
25. Yasuno F, Suhara T, Ichimiya T, et al. Decreased 5-HT1A receptor binding in amygdala of schizophrenia. Biol Psychiatry 2004;55(5):439–44.
26. Wilson AA, McCormick P, Kapur S, et al. Radiosynthesis and evaluation of [11C]-(+)-4-propyl-3,4,4a,5,6,10b-hexahydro-2H-naphtho[1,2-b][1,4]oxazin-9-ol as a potential radiotracer for in vivo imaging of the dopamine D2 high-affinity state with positron emission tomography. J Med Chem 2005;48(12): 4153–60.
27. Rabiner EA, Slifstein M, Nobrega J, et al. In vivo quantification of regional dopamine-D3 receptor binding potential of (+)-PHNO: studies in non-human primates and transgenic mice. Synapse 2009;63(9):782–93.
28. Boileau I, Guttman M, Rusjan P, et al. Decreased binding of the D3 dopamine receptor-preferring ligand [11C]-(+)-PHNO in drug-naive Parkinson's disease. Brain 2009;132(Pt 5):1366–75.
29. Lundkvist C, Sandell J, Någren K, et al. Improved syntheses of the PET radioligands, [11C]FLB 457, [11C]MDL 100907 and [11C]-CIT-FE, by the use of [11C]methyl triflate. J Labelled Comp Radiopharm 1998;41(6):545–56.
30. Någren K, Halldin C, Müller L, et al. Comparison of [11C]methyl triflate and [11C]methyl iodide in the synthesis of PET radioligands such as [11C][beta]-CIT and [11C][beta]-CFT. Nucl Med Biol 1995; 22(8):965–70.
31. Någren K, Müller L, Halldin C, et al. Improved synthesis of some commonly used PET radioligands by the use of [11C]methyl triflate. Nucl Med Biol 1995;22(2):235–9.
32. Mathis CA, Bacskai BJ, Kajdasz ST, et al. A lipophilic thioflavin-T derivative for positron emission tomography (PET) imaging of amyloid in brain. Bioorg Med Chem Lett 2002;12(3):295–8.
33. Mathis CA, Wang Y, Holt DP, et al. Synthesis and evaluation of 11C-labeled 6-substituted 2-arylbenzothiazoles as amyloid imaging agents. J Med Chem 2003;46(13):2740–54.
34. Wilson AA, Garcia A, Chestakova A, et al. A rapid one-step radiosynthesis of the beta-amyloid imaging radiotracer N-methyl-[11C]2-(4-methylaminophenyl)-6-hydroxybenzothiazole ([11C]-6-OH-BTA-1). J Labelled Comp Radiopharm 2004; 47(10):679–82.
35. Solbach C, Uebele M, Reischl G, et al. Efficient radiosynthesis of carbon-11 labelled uncharged thioflavin T derivatives using [11C]methyl triflate for [beta]-amyloid imaging in Alzheimer's disease with PET. Appl Radiat Isot 2005;62(4):591–5.
36. Klunk WE, Engler H, Nordberg A, et al. Imaging brain amyloid in Alzheimer's disease with Pittsburgh Compound-B. Ann Neurol 2004;55(3):306–19.
37. Haka MS, Kilbourn MR, Watkins GL, et al. Aryltrimethylammonium trifluoromethanesulfonates as precursors to aryl [18F]fluorides: improved synthesis of [18F]GBR-13119. J Labelled Comp Radiopharm 1989;27(7):823–33.

38. Kilbourn MR. Fluorine-18 labeling of radiopharmaceuticals. Nuclear science series, vol. NAS-NS-3203. Washington, DC: National Academy Press; 1990. 149.
39. Shiue CY, Fowler JS, Wolf AP, et al. No-carrier-added fluorine-18-labeled N-methylspiroperidol: synthesis and biodistribution in mice. J Nucl Med 1986; 27(2):226–34.
40. Wang GJ, Volkow ND, Logan J, et al. Evaluation of age-related changes in serotonin 5-HT2 and dopamine D2 receptor availability in healthy human subjects. Life Sci 1995;56(14):PL249–53.
41. Ding YS, Gatley SJ, Fowler JS, et al. Mapping nicotinic acetylcholine receptors with PET. Synapse 1996;24(4):403–7.
42. Horti A, Ravert HT, London ED, et al. Synthesis of a radiotracer for studying nicotinic acetylcholine receptors: (+/−)-exo-2-(2-[18F]fluoro-5-pyridyl)-7-azabicyclo[2.2.1]heptane. J Labelled Comp Radiopharm 1996;38(4):355–65.
43. Dolle F, Dolci L, Valette H, et al. Synthesis and nicotinic acetylcholine receptor in vivo binding properties of 2-fluoro-3-[2(S)-2-azetidinylmethoxy]pyridine: a new positron emission tomography ligand for nicotinic receptors. J Med Chem 1999;42(12):2251–9.
44. Ding YS, Liang F, Fowler JS, et al. Synthesis of [18F]norchlorofluoroepibatidine and its N-methyl derivative: new PET ligands for mapping nicotinic acetylcholine receptors. J Labelled Comp Radiopharm 1997;39(10):827–32.
45. Block D, Coenen HH, Stöcklin G. The N.C.A. nucleophilic 18F-fluorination of 1,N-disubstituted alkanes as fluoroalkylation agents. J Labelled Comp Radiopharm 1987;24(9):1029–42.
46. Moerlein SM, Perlmutter JS. Binding of 5-(2′-[18F]fluoroethyl)flumazenil to central benzodiazepine receptors measured in living baboon by positron emission tomography. Eur J Pharmacol 1992;218(1):109–15.
47. Mach RH, Elder ST, Morton TE, et al. The use of [18F]4-fluorobenzyl iodide (FBI) in PET radiotracer synthesis: model alkylation studies and its application in the design of dopamine D1 and D2 receptor-based imaging agents. Nucl Med Biol 1993;20(6):777–94.
48. Hatano K, Ido T, Iwata R. The synthesis of o- and p-[18F]fluorobenzyl bromides and their application to the prepatation of labeled neuroleptics. J Labelled Comp Radiopharm 1991;29(4):373–80.
49. Ravert HT, Madar I, Dannals RF. Radiosynthesis of 3-[18F]fluoropropyl and 4-[18F]fluorobenzyl triarylphosphonium ions. J Labelled Comp Radiopharm 2004;47(8):469–76.
50. Marik J, Sutcliffe JL. Click for PET: rapid preparation of [18F]fluoropeptides using CuI catalyzed 1,3-dipolar cycloaddition. Tetrahedron Lett 2006;47(37):6681–4.
51. Glaser M, Arstad E. "Click labeling" with 2-[18f]fluoroethylazide for positron emission tomography. Bioconjug Chem 2007;18(3):989–93.
52. Kuhnast B, Hinnen F, Tavitian B, et al. [^{18}F]FPyKYNE, a fluoropyridine-based alkyne reagent designed for the fluorine-18
labelling of macromolecules using click chemistry. J Labelled Comp Radiopharm 2008;51(9):336–42.
53. Inkster JA, Guérin B, Ruth TJ, et al. Radiosynthesis and bioconjugation of [^{18}F]FPy5yne, a prosthetic group for the ^{18}F labeling of bioactive peptides. J Labelled Comp Radiopharm 2008;51(14):444–52.
54. Thonon D, Kech CC, Paris JRM, et al. New strategy for the preparation of clickable peptides and labeling with 1-(azidomethyl)-4-[^{18}F]-fluorobenzene for PET. Bioconjug Chem 2009;20(4):817–23.
55. Glaser M, Robins EG. "Click labelling" in PET radiochemistry. J Labelled Comp Radiopharm 2009; 52(10):407–14.
56. Nickles RJ, Daube ME, Ruth TJ. An $^{18}O_2$ target for the production of [^{18}F]F_2. Int J Appl Radiat Isot 1984;35(2):117–22.
57. Chirakal R, Firnau G, Garnett ES. High yield synthesis of 6-[18F]fluoro-L-dopa. J Nucl Med 1986;27(3):417–21.
58. Chirakal R, Schrobilgen GJ, Firnau G, et al. Synthesis of 18F labelled fluoro-m-tyrosine, fluoro-m-tyramine and fluoro-3-hydroxyphenylacetic acid. Int J Rad Appl Instrum A 1991;42(2):113–9.
59. Bergman J, Lehikoinen P, Solin O. Specific radioactivity and radiochemical yield in electrophilic fluorination: case study with [18F]CFT. J Labelled Comp Radiopharm 1997;40(S):38–9.
60. Komar G, Seppanen M, Eskola O, et al. 18F-EF5: a new PET tracer for imaging hypoxia in head and neck cancer. J Nucl Med 2008;49(12):1944–51.
61. Bergman J, Solin O. Fluorine-18-labeled fluorine gas for synthesis of tracer molecules. Nucl Med Biol 1997;24(7):677–83.
62. Ametamey SM, Honer M, Schubiger PA. Molecular imaging with PET. Chem Rev 2008;108(5): 1501–16.
63. Hansch C, Leo A, Hoekman D. Exploring QSAR: hydrophobic, electronic, and steric constants. In: Heller SR, editor, In: Computer applications in chemistry books, vol. 2. Washington, DC: American Chemical Society; 1995. p. 348.
64. Nagai Y, Obayashi S, Ando K, et al. Progressive changes of pre- and post-synaptic dopaminergic biomarkers in conscious MPTP-treated cynomolgus monkeys measured by positron emission tomography. Synapse 2007;61(10):809–19.
65. Doudet DJ, Miyake H, Finn RT, et al. 6-18F-L-dopa imaging of the dopamine neostriatal system in normal and clinically normal MPTP-treated rhesus monkeys. Exp Brain Res 1989;78(1):69–80.
66. Shively CA, Grant KA, Ehrenkaufer RL, et al. Social stress, depression, and brain dopamine in female cynomolgus monkeys. Ann N Y Acad Sci 1997; 807:574–7.

67. Nader MA, Czoty PW, Gould RW, et al. Review. Positron emission tomography imaging studies of dopamine receptors in primate models of addiction. Philos Trans R Soc Lond, B, Biol Sci 2008; 363(1507):3223–32.
68. Voytko ML, Mach RH, Gage HD, et al. Cholinergic activity of aged rhesus monkeys revealed by positron emission tomography. Synapse 2001;39(1):95–100.
69. VanBrocklin HF. Radiopharmaceuticals for drug development: United States regulatory perspective current radiopharmaceuticals 2008;1(1):2–6.
70. Ido T, Wan CN, Fowler JS, et al. Fluorination with molecular fluorine. A convenient synthesis of 2-deoxy-2-fluoro-D-glucose. J Org Chem 1977; 42(13):2341–2.
71. Proposed rule (21 CFR Part 212): current good manufacturing practice for positron emission tomography drugs. Fed Regist 2005;70(181):55038–62.
72. Draft guidance on current good manufacturing practice for positron emission tomography drug products; Availability. Fed Regist 2005;70(181):55145.
73. Radiopharmaceuticals for positron emission tomography: compounding. The United States Pharmacopeia and National Formulary USP 32 -NF 27. Rockville (MD): The United States Pharmacopeia Convention, Inc; 2009. Chapter 823.
74. Current good manufacturing practice for positron emission tomography drugs. Fed Regist 2009; 74(236):65409–36.
75. Innovation or stagnation: challenge and opportunity on the critical path to new medical products FDA challenges and opportunities report [internet communication]. March 2004. Available at: http://www.fda.gov/ScienceResearch/SpecialTopics/CriticalPathInitiative/CriticalPathOpportunitiesReports/ucm077262.htm. Accessed October 4, 2009.
76. FDA guidance for industry, investigators and reviewers: exploratory IND studies [internet communication]. January 2006. Available at. http://www.fda.gov/downloads/Drugs/GuidanceCompliance-RegulatoryInformation/Guidances/UCM078933.pdf. Accessed October 4, 2009.
77. Position paper on non-clinical safety studies to support clinical trials with a single microdose: CPMP/SWP/2599/2502/Rev2591. London (UK): Committee for Medicinal Products for Human Use (CHP), European Medicines Agency; 2004. Available at: www.emea.europa.eu/pdfs/human/swp/259902en.pdf. Accessed October 4, 2009.
78. Residual solvents/organic volatile impurities. The United States Pharmacopeia and National Formulary. USP 32-NF 27. Rockville (MD): The United States Pharmacopeia Convention, Inc; 2009. Chapter 467.
79. Mock BH, Winkle W, Vavrek MT. A color spot test for the detection of Kryptofix 2.2.2 in [18F]FDG preparations. Nucl Med Biol 1997;24(2):193–5.
80. Pharmaceutical compounding—sterile preparations. The United States Pharmacopeia and National Formulary. USP 32-NF 27. Rockville (MD): The United States Pharmacopeia Convention, Inc; 2009. Chapter 797.

Structure-Function–Based Quantitative Brain Image Analysis

Habib Zaidi, PhD, PD[a,b,*], Marie-Louise Montandon, PhD[a],
Frédéric Assal, MD[c]

KEYWORDS

- Image fusion • PET-MRI • Quantification
- Neurodegenerative disease • Structural brain imaging
- Molecular brain imaging • PET • MRI

Modern functional brain mapping techniques, such as PET, single-photon emission CT (SPECT), functional MRI (fMRI), electroencephalography, magnetoencephalography, optical imaging, and neuroanatomic tools, have been used for assessing the functional organization of the human brain.[1,2] Through these techniques, neuroscience has progressed to a great extent in the understanding of the brain in health and disease. A comprehensive overview of these techniques and associated technologies is beyond the scope of this review, which focuses on recently developed high-resolution PET systems and dual-modality PET-MR units dedicated for brain imaging, particularly in the context of the assessment of dementia and related disorders.

The tendency in MR instrumentation development is to go for higher field strength to increase the signal-to-noise ratio in the resulting MRIs and as such achieving the highest possible field strength was strived for.[3] Although 3 T is becoming the state-of-the-art for clinical MRI, ultra–high-field MR systems are receiving considerable attention in preclinical[4] and clinical brain research. Several 7-T commercial scanners have become operational[5] whereas experimental 8- and 9.4-T scanners are under investigation.[6] Alternatively, the demand for functional, metabolic, and molecular imaging of the brain[7] has stimulated the development of dedicated high-resolution PET systems.[8,9]

To respond to the requirements of emerging clinical and research applications of correlated anatomic and functional brain imaging, several innovative developments in high performance standalone (PET and MRI) and dual-modality imaging instrumentation combining modalities have been proposed or are currently under design or testing. The development of combined PET-MR systems allowing simultaneous or sequential PET and MR brain imaging is an active research area.[10,11] This article discusses recent advances in multimodality brain imaging and the role of correlative fusion imaging and advanced quantitative imaging procedures in the clinical setting. Future opportunities and challenges facing the adoption of multimodality brain imaging also are addressed.

NEUROIMAGING IN THE DIAGNOSIS OF DEMENTIA AND RELATED DISORDERS

Neuroimaging is recommended by the 2001 practice parameters of the American Academy of

This work was supported by the Swiss National Science Foundation under grants SNSF 31003A-125246 and SNSF 33CM30-124114.

[a] Division of Nuclear Medicine, Geneva University Hospital, Geneva CH-1211, Switzerland
[b] Geneva Neuroscience Center, Geneva University, Geneva CH-1211, Switzerland
[c] Neurology, Department of Clinical Neurosciences, Geneva University Hospital, Geneva CH-1211, Switzerland
* Corresponding author. Division of Nuclear Medicine, Geneva University Hospital, Geneva CH-1211, Switzerland.
E-mail address: habib.zaidi@hcuge.ch

PET Clin 5 (2010) 155–168
doi:10.1016/j.cpet.2010.02.003
1556-8598/10/$ – see front matter

Neurology in the setting of neurodegenerative dementia and related disorders.[12] Structural brain imaging, preferably using MRI, not only rules out strokes, chronic subdural hematomas, cerebral neoplasms, or normal pressure hydrocephalus but also reveals characteristic patterns of regional atrophy that are commonly associated with clinical diagnosis.

In Alzheimer disease (AD), most investigators focused on reduced volume in the hippocampus or entorhinal cortex,[13–19] although its usefulness compared with clinical assessment alone has been questioned.[20] Other MRI-based studies reported atrophy in the superior parietal cortex and posterior cingulate/precuneus.[21–25] In frontotemporal dementia (FTD), atrophy is predominant in frontotemporal regions, depending on the clinical phenotype (ie, bilateral medial frontal or right frontal in the behavioral variant, left inferior frontal/left insula in the progressive nonfluent aphasia variant, and anterior temporal in the semantic dementia variant).[26–30]

Structural neuroimaging is less specific in the diagnosis of other non-AD neurodegenerative dementias and related disorders. Hippocampal atrophy is present in Lewy body dementia (LBD) and Parkinson disease dementia but to a lesser degree than in AD.[19,31–34] Predominant asymetric frontoparietal and midbrain atrophy is found, respectively, in corticobasal degeneration (CBD) and supranuclear palsy (PSP).[35–37]

Although not recommended by the 2001 practice parameters of the American Academy of Neurology, functional brain PET imaging using [^{18}F]-fluorodeoxyglucose (FDG)[38,39] and amyloid plaque tracers (mostly ^{11}C-labeled Pittsburgh compound B)[40] are increasingly used in the diagnosis of most common dementias.[41] The latter is still under investigation and not widely available for clinical use.

In AD, FDG-PET reveals hypometabolism in the precuneus/posterior cingulate and the lateral parietotemporal cortex[42–45] with sensitivity of 93% and specificity of 76%.[46] FDG-PET may be useful in distinguishing AD from FTD[47,48] or from vascular dementia.[49] Amyloid PET tracers may also help to discriminate early AD or mild cognitive impairment from normal controls,[50–52] and AD from FTD.[53,54] In FTD, FDG-PET supports the diagnosis but is not part of the Neary criteria.[55] It might be more sensitive than structural MRI in its early stages because hypometabolism in the frontotemporal regions may precede atrophy.[56,57]

In LBD, FDG-PET studies demonstrated parietotemporal and occipital hypoactivity[48,58–61] and low dopaminergic activity in the striatum using dopamine transporter imaging with ^{123}I-FP-CIT SPECT.[62,63] In CBD and PSP, when compared with each other or to controls, the former exhibited asymmetric hypometabolism in frontoparietal regions and lenticular nuclei whereas the latter exhibited asymmetric hypometabolism in frontal cortex, thalamus, and midbrain.[64–67] Nevertheless, currently available studies, often based on longitudinal changes over time, primarily evaluate structural and metabolic changes in groups of patients and are often inadequate to rely upon when evaluating individual patients.

Diagnosis of main dementias and related disorders at an early stage remains a challenge because of overlaps not only between main clinical diagnosis but also with normal aging.[68] Additional carefully designed clinical trials are needed to better validate structural MRI and FDG-PET (and other probes) as a diagnostic biomarker. Several studies have focused on correlated structural and functional data analysis involving coregistration of multimodality images. In AD, the hypoactivity in the posterior cingulate and in the precuneus remained significant after partial volume effect (PVE) correction using FDG-PET,[69–72] although other investigators suggested that the hypometabolism in the precuneus could at least be partly explained by the regional atrophy.[73] This discordance between atrophy and hypometabolism was present at the predementia stage where posterior cingulate/precuneus hypometabolism was associated with early memory deficits and left temporal hypometabolism marked the conversion to AD.[74] In LBD, FDG-PET findings report significant hypometabolism in the temporal, parietal, occipital, and frontal areas compared with those in the normal control group.[60]

OVERVIEW OF DEDICATED INSTRUMENTATION FOR MULTIMODALITY BRAIN IMAGING

Fig. 1 highlights the historical developments of brain PET imaging showing the improvement in image quality and spatial resolution as consequence of the noticeable improvement in PET instrumentation and image reconstruction techniques. As in whole-body imaging, high-detection sensitivity and spatial resolution and high-contrast and contrast resolution are the main concerns for imaging system design and constitute the basic requirements to achieving appropriate levels of image quality and quantitative accuracy. Thus, different dedicated brain PET designs have been and are still being developed in academic and corporate settings, with only a few units offered commercially. More recently, advanced versions of these technologies have begun to be used in

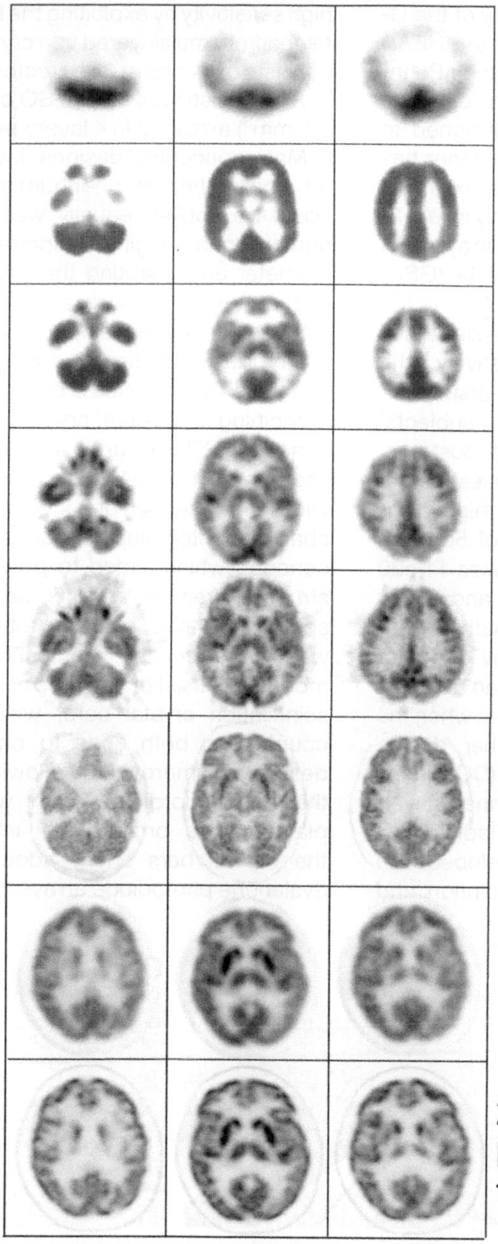

Fig. 1. Illustration of the significant improvement in clinical FDG brain PET image quality and spatial resolution resulting from the improvement in scanner performance for each generation during the past 3 decades. (*Reproduced from* Siemens Medical Solutions, Knoxville, TN; with permission.)

the study of brain function in myriad clinical and experimental settings.

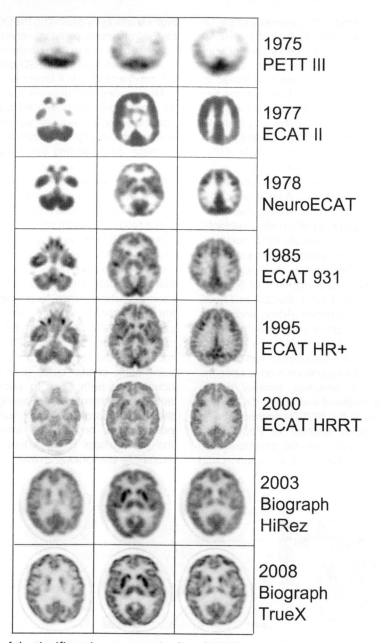

To meet the objectives set by the molecular neuroimaging community, new-generation, high-resolution, 3D-only brain PET tomographs have been designed.[8,9] Current existing commercial brain PET technology (eg, the ECAT–high-resolution research tomograph [HRRT] developed by CTI-Siemens[75]) and other dedicated prototype designs, including G-PET[76] (developed at the University of Pennsylvania) and the Hamamatsu SHR-12000,[77] constitute state-of-the-art high resolution PET instrumentation dedicated for brain research. The HRRT consists of octagonal arrangements (42.4 cm face to face) of phoswich scintillator block detectors made of 2 layers of 64 small lutetium oxyorthosilicate (LSO) crystals (each 2.1 $\times$ 2.1 $\times$ 7.5 mm^3) with 2 different decay times ($\Delta\tau$ ~7 ns). The crystals (15 mm total active length) are oriented normal to the octagon sides, hence essentially pointing in radial direction. The geometry of the G-PET brain scanner is similar to that of the HEAD PENN-PET[78] (developed at the University of Pennsylvania); however, the detector technology and electronic components have been redesigned to achieve improved performance. This scanner has a detector ring diameter of 42 cm and an axial field of view (FOV) of 25.6 cm and operates only in fully 3-D mode. It comprises 18,560 (320 × 58 array) 4 × 4 × 10 mm^3 gadolinium samarium oxalate (GSO) crystals coupled through a continuous light guide to 288 (36 × 8 array) 39-mm photomultiplier tubes in a hexagonal arrangement. Alternatively, the gantry and bed motions of the Hamamatsu SHR-12000 were designed specifically to allow subjects' scanning in lying, sitting, and standing postures, thus giving the possibility to research investigators of performing activation studies with high flexibility.[77] This scanner has a diameter of 50.8 cm and an axial FOV of 16.3 cm. It comprises 11,520 crystals arranged in 24 detector rings and 8 × 4 (2.8 × 6.55 × 30 mm^3 per crystal) bismuth germanate (BGO) detector blocks readout by compact position-sensitive PMTs. The scanner can be operated in 2-D or 3-D data acquisition modes when the interplane septa are retracted. Another design providing 4-layer depth-of-interaction (DOI) information, referred to as the jPET-D4 scanner (developed at the National Institute of Radiological Sciences, Chiba, Japan), was also developed with the aim of achieving high spatial resolution and high sensitivity by exploiting the DOI information obtained from multilayered thin crystals.[79] The system consists of 5 rings of 24 detector blocks each, each block consisting of 1024 GSO crystals (2.9 × 2.9 × 7.5 mm^3) arranged in 4 layers of 16 × 16 arrays.

Many conceptual designs developed specifically for small animal and nonhuman primates imaging could be applied equally well to high-resolution human brain imaging by increasing detector ring diameter and adapting the detector components accordingly. One such example is the clearPET Neuro scanner (developed by the Crystal Clear collaboration) dedicated for nonhuman primates imaging,[80] which uses a phoswich detector block combining 2 10-mm crystal layers of lutetium-based (LSO:Ce and LuYAP:Ce) scintillators segmented into 64 (8 × 8) detection elements with a cross section of 2 × 2 mm^2 coupled to multichannel photomultiplier tubes. The axial brain PET concept, which aimed to provide full 3-D reconstruction free of parallax errors with excellent spatial resolution over the total detector volume, was also recently suggested.[81] The detector modules consist of matrices of long axially oriented scintillation crystal bars, which are individually coupled on both ends to photodetectors. This design was improved by allowing the derivation of the axial coordinate from wavelength shifting plastic strips orthogonally interleaved between the crystal bars and readout by Geiger-mode avalanche photodiode arrays.[82]

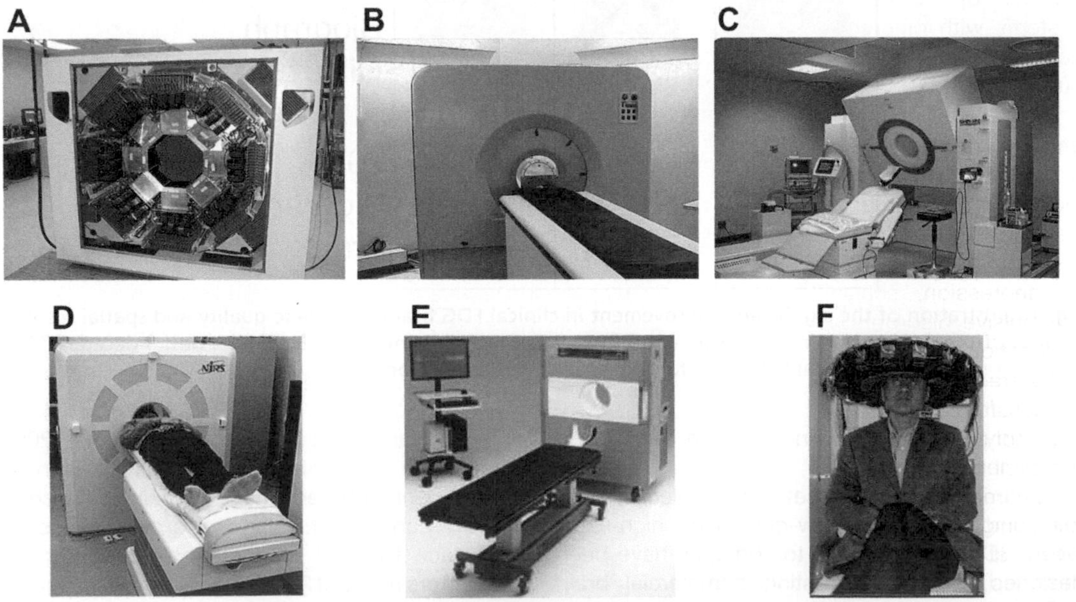

Fig. 2. Photographs of dedicated brain PET scanners showing (*A*) the HRRT camera based on LSO scintillation crystals and the phoswich concept, (*B*) the GSO-based PET (G-PET) camera, (*C*) the Hamamatsu SHR-12,000 PET scanner based on BGO detector blocks, (*D*) the jPET-D4 brain PET scanner, (*E*) the NeuroPET, and (*F*) the PET-Hat wearable PET system.

More recently, a novel platform, the NeuroPET (PhotoDetection Systems Inc, Boxboro, MA, USA), was proposed and made commercially available.[83] The Rat Conscious Animal PET (RATCAP; developed at Brookhaven National Laboratory, Upton, NY, USA)—a complete 3-D tomograph designed to image the brain of an awake rat,[84] like the PET-Hat (developed at Kobe City College of Technology, Kobe, Japan) wearable PET system—was also recently developed.[85] Because semiconductor detectors usually have higher-energy resolution compared with scintillation crystals. A new semiconductor-based brain PET scanner using a DOI detection system to reduce parallax error, thus achieving high spatial resolution and reduced scatter fraction, was proposed.[86] **Fig. 2** shows photographs of the some of the designs.

Few studies focused on the comparative assessment of the resulting spatial resolution and quantitative accuracy of brain imaging using dedicated high-resolution brain scanners with conventional whole-body designs. Although the Biograph 6 (Siemens Medical Solutions) PET-CT system was reported to have similar performance characteristics as the HR+ (Siemens Medical Solutions) for neuroimaging studies,[87] the higher pharmacokinetic parameter estimates obtained from the HRRT versus ECAT-HR+ (both manufactured by Siemens Medical Solutions) PET studies indicate improved HRRT PET quantification primarily due to a reduction in PVE.[88] This raises the issue of transfer of normal databases between PET systems with different performance characteristics for which some solutions have been suggested.

The availability of correlated functional (PET) and anatomic images (MRI) was exploited in a variety of clinical neurologic applications, including for cerebrovascular disorders, brain trauma, stroke, epilepsy, dementia, Parkinson disease, brain tumor, and mental disorders, such as depression, schizophrenia, and obsessive-compulsive disorders, as well as for localization of functional neuroactivation detected with PET. Software-based image registration has been successfully applied to neurologic studies (particularly for nonspecific tracers, such as FDG), where the skull provides a rigid structure that maintains the geometric relationship of structures within the brain and are now used routinely for clinical procedures at most institutions.[89,90] Although such methods are fully automated, their performance depends on many physiologic and technical aspects; further research is being conducted to evaluate their suitability in different clinical situations and their potential use in motion correction frequently encountered during lengthy PET scanning protocols.[91]

Contrary to hardware-based hybrid imaging combining PET and CT (PET-CT) systems in a single gantry to allow sequential scanning, which was successfully introduced in clinics in the beginning of this decade, combining PET with MR to allow simultaneous acquisition of spatially and temporally correlated PET-MR data sets is technically more challenging owing to the strong magnetic fields in the MR subsystem. The history of combined PET-MR dates back to the mid-1990s, however, before the advent of PET-CT.[92] Despite the challenges and technical difficulties, a clinical PET-MR prototype (BrainPET, Siemens Medical Solutions) dedicated for simultaneous PET-MR brain imaging was developed and installed in a few institutions for validation and testing.[10] **Fig. 3** illustrates the conceptual design and photograph of the integrated MR/PET scanner showing isocentric layering of MR head coil, PET detector ring, and MR magnet tunnel together with concurrently acquired clinical MR, PET, and fused MR/PET images. The system is being assessed in a clinical setting by exploiting the full potential of anatomic MRI in terms of high, soft tissue contrast sensitivity in addition to the many other possibilities offered by this modality, including blood oxygenation level–dependent imaging, fMRI, diffusion-weighted imaging, perfusion-weighted imaging, and diffusion tensor imaging.[93] A second sequential combined PET-MR system was also designed for molecular-genetic brain imaging by docking separate PET and MR systems together so that they share a common bed, which passes through the FOV of both cameras.[11] This is achieved by combining 2 high-end imaging devices, the HRRT and a 7-T MRI with submillimeter resolution.

QUANTITATIVE ANALYSIS OF BRAIN PET DATA

Subjective qualitative visual interpretation or semi-quantitative analysis approaches involving operator-dependent and time-consuming manual volume-of-interest delineation techniques have been performed for decades and still are used routinely in many nuclear medicine departments. In the past few years, however, spatial normalization (or anatomic standardization) methods have become popular and widely available, thus allowing voxel-based analysis to be made. This has had an enormous contribution to PET activation studies and other studies involving the assessment of functional changes associated with neuropathology. Anatomic standardization allows the

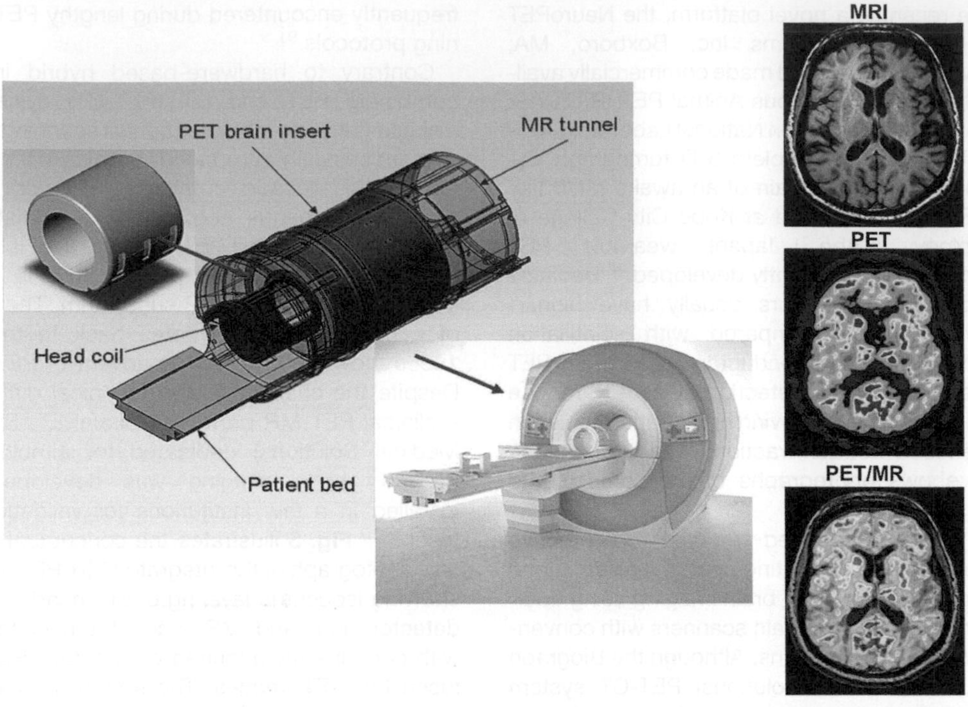

Fig. 3. Drawing and photograph of integrated MR/PET design showing isocentric layering of MR head coil, PET detector ring, and MR magnet tunnel (*left*). Simultaneously acquired MR, PET, and fused combined MRI/PET images of a 66-year-old man after intravenous injection of 370 MBq of FDG. Tracer distribution was recorded for 20 minutes at steady state after 120 minutes (*right*). (*Adapted and reprinted from* Schlemmer HP, Pichler BJ, Schmand M, et al. Simultaneous MR/PET imaging of the human brain: feasibility study. Radiology 2008;248:1028–35; with permission.)

transformation of brain images of individual subjects into a standard coordinate system, such as the stereotactic coordinate system proposed by Talairach and Tournoux.[94] Several methods for spatial normalization of brain images have been reported in the scientific literature, including Human Brain Atlas,[95] Statistical Parametric Mapping (SPM) software package (Wellcome Trust Centre for Neuroimaging, UCL Institute of Neurology, University College London, London, United Kingdom),[96] and 3D Stereotactic-Surface Projections (SSP) method developed by Minoshima and colleagues.[97]

The Human Brain Atlas uses morphologic information provided by PET-registered MRI.[95] The accuracy of the method is limited, however, by the precision that can be achieved by the coregistration procedure used to realign PET and MRI. SPM is among the state-of-the-art packages for statistical analysis of neuroimaging data including PET, SPECT, and fMRI. It is well documented, freely available, technically supported by well-established brain imaging centers,[96] and widely used by the neuroimaging community. The technique relies on morphologic images for the transformation into a standard coordinate system and has been extensively used to distinguish which structures of the brain are significantly activated by a neuroactivation task for a group of subjects or to identify which areas of the brain present with significant differences in metabolism (or cerebral blood flow) when comparing patient images with those of healthy volunteers. The steps involved in the statistical analysis of brain images include (1) spatial normalization of brain images into a standard stereotactic space for subsequent voxel-based analyses, (2) gaussian smoothing to correct for interindividual differences in underlying brain structures and allow the application of the general linear model approach for consecutive statistical analysis, and (2) the construction of statistical parametric maps.

Originally, SPM was developed for PET activation studies on healthy volunteers and was not intended for clinical application to diseased brains. For this reason, NEUROSTAT (Department of Internal Medicine, University of Michigan, Ann Arbor, MI, USA) was specially designed for statistical comparison between a normal database and diseased brains presenting with focal metabolic (perfusion) lesions.[97] The technique projects the cortical activity visualized in a 3-D volume image onto the brain surface to generate a surface representation of the cortical activity distribution. This method was combined with the previously proposed standardization method by the same group, and the entire process referred to as 3D-SSP NEUROSTAT.

Among the commercial software packages, Brain Registration and Automated SPECT Semi-quantification (BRASS) (Nuclear Diagnostics, Hägersted, Sweden) was designed for routine clinical brain SPECT and PET applications and allows 2 complementary quantitative comparisons of patient images with a 3-D reference atlas created from images of healthy volunteers: (1) a voxel-wise method and (2) an ROI-based regional analysis. The first can distinguish small defects but is sensitive to small registration errors and to the quality of the template whereas the second determines the mean and *z* scores within 3-D regions defined by a region map that has been matched to the template.[98] **Fig. 4** illustrates transverse views of an FDG-PET image of a patient with probable AD. The 3-D anatomically standardized brain PET template, the quantified defect for this patient, and the *z* score image obtained by the automated BRASS quantification procedure are also shown. PMOD (PMOD Technologies, Zürich, Switzerland) is another popular commercial multimodality medical imaging package based on a large FDG database of normal subjects acquired in a multicenter trial[99] for the discrimination between AD and controls. The PMOD Alzheimer discrimination analysis tool is an authorized implementation of this methodology. This method, although not approved for clinical use, may be used to analyze FDG-PET scans of patients with suspected AD for automatic discrimination analysis. The results point out brain areas with significant uptake

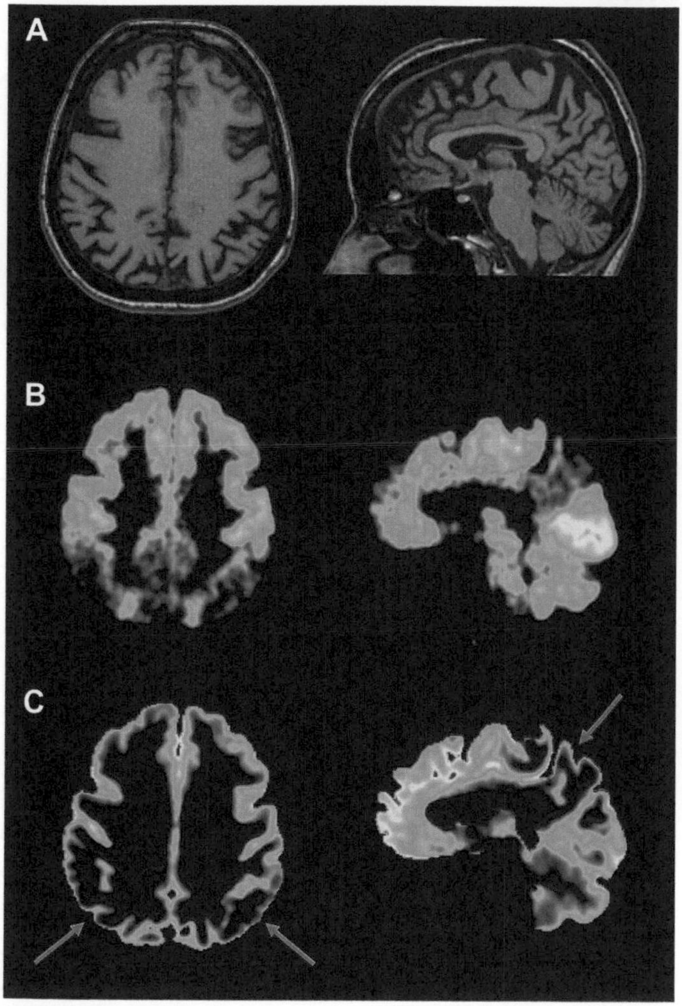

Fig. 4. Illustration of MRI-guided PVE correction impact in functional brain PET imaging showing for a patient with probable AD the original T1-weighted MRI (*A*) and PET images before (*B*) and after (*C*) PVE correction. The arrows point to evidence that the hypometabolism extends beyond the atrophy.

reduction ($P<.05$) and indicate a criterion of scan abnormality together with its error probability.

Several neuroimaging studies have been performed with the aim of evaluating the functional changes in healthy elderly brains and in patients with neurodegenerative diseases. The accurate measurement of tracer concentration, however, is corrupted by various physical degrading factors, including positron range,[100] limited spatial resolution and resulting PVE,[101] contribution from scattered photons,[102] photon attenuation,[103] patient motion,[104] and the image reconstruction algorithm.[105] Attenuation of photons degrades the visual quality and quantitative accuracy of PET images, thereby adversely affecting qualitative interpretation and quantitation of activity concentration. Accurate attenuation correction is, therefore, mandatory in quantitative PET image reconstruction and plays a pivotal role in clinical PET scanning protocols.[103] PVE leads to underestimation of the activity concentration in small structures of the brain (ie, with dimensions smaller than approximately 2–4 times the full width at half maximum of the scanner's point spread function). This problem is accentuated in the presence of brain atrophy, such as that encountered in AD, where this diluting effect is more pronounced. Compensation for PVE is then mandatory to offer the possibility of distinguishing the loss of radiotracer uptake due to PVE from the true metabolic values that decline with age or neuropathology.[69,106]

PVE compensation usually involves the following steps: (1) characterization of the point spread function of the imaging system, (2) characterization of the tissue components that participate in the uptake and metabolism of the tracer, and (3) characterization of the resolution effects in terms of correction factors or maps. PVE correction methods in brain PET may or may not require

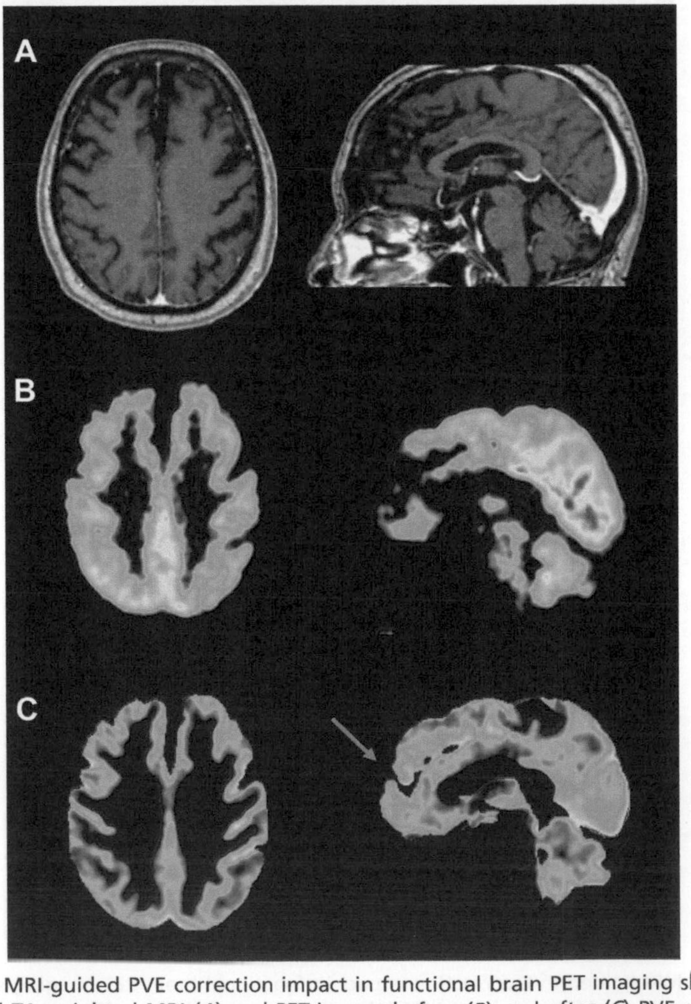

Fig. 5. Illustration of MRI-guided PVE correction impact in functional brain PET imaging showing for a patient with FTD the original T1-weighted MRI (*A*) and PET images before (*B*) and after (*C*) PVE correction. The arrow points to evidence that the hypometabolism matches the atrophy.

the availability of additional structural information from MRI of the same subject. MRI-guided PVE correction algorithms require as input segmented MRIs coregistered to PET data. It is assumed, therefore, that each segment of the activity distribution model represents a distinct and homogeneous activity distribution. Variants of this class of algorithms have been suggested and implemented successfully in a growing number of research studies.[101] Popular voxel-based approaches consider a heterogeneous distribution of the tracer uptake using a more realistic anatomic mask derived from MRI that makes the distinction between gray matter (GM) and white matter (WM) to account for WM activity contribution to measurements of GM activity concentration.[107,108]

The general principle of voxel-based MR-guided PVE correction in brain PET imaging involves the following steps[108]: first, the MRIs and PET images are spatially realigned, and then, the MRI is segmented into WM and GM. The latter is a popular research topic and a variety of image segmentation tools are available and have been used for this purpose.[109,110] The next step involves convolving the segmented WM and GM images by the PET scanner's spatial resolution modeled by a gaussian response function. The GM PET image is subsequently obtained by subtraction of the simulated WM PET image from the original PET image coregistered to MRI. The PVE corrected GM PET image is then obtained by dividing the GM PET image by the convolved GM MRI. A binary mask for GM is finally applied. Alternative approaches using deconvolution[111] and structural-functional synergetic multiresolution analysis[112,113] as well as those incorporated in statistical iterative reconstruction techniques,[114] which are more robust to coregistration errors, are being explored and exploited in research investigations.

CLINICAL IMPLICATIONS OF CORRELATED STRUCTURAL-FUNCTION–BASED QUANTITATIVE ANALYSIS

In recent years, efforts have been made to understand brain structure and function as they are related to aging and especially to neurodegenerative disorders. Multimodality brain imaging might

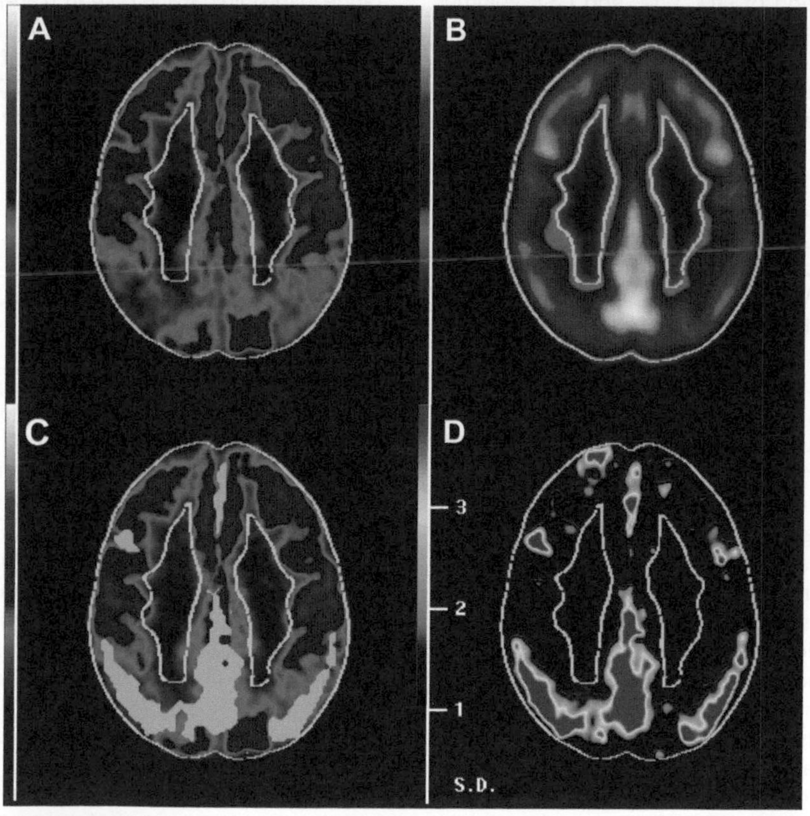

Fig. 6. Transverse views of the FDG-PET image of a patient with probable AD (*A*), the PET template (*B*), the quantified defect for this patient (*C*), and the *z*-score image (*D*), where the large red region indicates a region of significant hypometabolism. The isocontour indicates the external outline of the template.

be extremely important in the setting of future drugs that may help decrease disease progression. A main concern has been related to the PVE correction for cerebral metabolism in the atrophied brain, particularly in AD. **Figs. 5** and **6** illustrate the impact of PVE correction in functional FDG-PET brain imaging of a patient with probable AD and another patient with probable FTD, respectively.[115] The voxel-based MRI-guided PVE correction used follows the approach by Matsuda and colleagues[108] (described previously). In the early 1990s, it was already reported in the scientific literature that, although whole-brain metabolism is significantly reduced in AD patients compared with control subjects, this decrease loses its significance when metabolic rates are corrected for atrophy.[69,116] These findings stipulate that the hypometabolism of AD patients is related to atrophy whereas the remaining cerebral tissue has a metabolism comparable with that in controls. More recently, Bural and colleagues[117] reported on a new method using an MRI-based segmentation technique allowing the calculation of the standardized uptake values (SUV) in the GM, WM, and cerebrospinal fluid (CSF) in the corresponding PET images. This approach consists of the calculation of GM, WM, and CSF volumes from the segmented MRI. The next step involves the computation of the mean SUV representing the whole metabolic activity of the brain from the FDG-PET images. The whole-brain volume is calculated by summing the GM, WM, and CSF volumes, which is then used to calculate the global cerebral metabolic activity by multiplying the mean SUV by the total brain volume. Likewise, the global WM metabolic activity is estimated by multiplying the mean SUV for the WM by the WM volume. The CSF metabolic activity is assumed to be nil. The global GM metabolic activity is estimated by subtracting the global WM metabolic activity from that of the whole brain, which is then divided by the GM volume to provide an accurate estimate of the SUV for GM compartment.[118]

Correlative multimodality imaging of the brain might be a new tool not only to better diagnose neurodegenerative dementias and related disorders in differential and early diagnosis but also to better understand structure-function relationship.[119] It might be postulated that mismatch between hypometabolism and atrophy would imply different neuronal mechanisms than absence of mismatch in terms of disease progression, cognitive reserve, and neuronal plasticity. In addition, it might be hypothesized that mismatch might precede atrophy/structural changes or suggest hypometabolism-inducing factors, such as disconnection, loss of synapses, or protein deposition. On the contrary, regions where atrophy and hypometabolism are matched may benefit from compensatory mechanisms, suggesting neural plasticity. More importantly, different patterns might emerge in the course of the disease in the same individual in response to pharmacologic treatment, cognitive training, or compensatory mechanisms.

SUMMARY

Neurodegenerative dementias and related disorders produce significant alterations in the brain that may not be detectable with neuropsychological tests or with structural imaging, in the case of early or presymptomatic stage of a disease, because of overlaps with normal aging, or that may not be disease-specific (ie, the frontal variant of AD and FTD). FDG-PET, which is widely available is therefore ideally suited for monitoring cell/molecular events in early stages of neurodegenerative diseases, as well as in differential diagnosis and during pharmacologic therapy for monitoring of treatment response. During the past 2 decades, molecular brain imaging using PET and MR has advanced elegantly and steadily gained importance in the clinical and research arenas. Software- and hardware-based multimodality brain imaging has enabled the implementation of sophisticated anatomic-guided quantitative PET procedures that undoubtedly will revolutionize clinical diagnosis and offer unique capabilities for the clinical neuroimaging community and neuroscience researchers at large.

REFERENCES

1. Gilman S. Imaging the brain. First of two parts. N Engl J Med 1998;338:812–20.
2. Hammoud DA, Hoffman JM, Pomper MG. Molecular neuroimaging: from conventional to emerging techniques. Radiology 2007;245:21–42.
3. Hu X, Norris DG. Advances in high-field magnetic resonance imaging. Annu Rev Biomed Eng 2004; 6:157–84.
4. Cudalbu C, Mlynarik V, Xin L, et al. Comparison of T1 relaxation times of the neurochemical profile in rat brain at 9.4 tesla and 14.1 tesla. Magn Reson Med 2009;62:862–7.
5. van der Zwaag W, Francis S, Head K, et al. fMRI at 1.5, 3 and 7 T: characterising BOLD signal changes. Neuroimage 2009;47:1425–34.
6. Atkinson IC, Renteria L, Burd H, et al. Safety of human MRI at static fields above the FDA 8 T guideline: sodium imaging at 9.4 T does not affect vital signs or cognitive ability. J Magn Reson Imaging 2007;26:1222–7.

7. Jacobs AH, Li H, Winkeler A, et al. PET-based molecular imaging in neuroscience. Eur J Nucl Med Mol Imaging 2003;30:1051–65.
8. Zaidi H, Montandon M-L. The new challenges of brain PET imaging technology. Curr Med Imaging Rev 2006;2:3–13.
9. Sossi V. Cutting-edge brain imaging with positron emission tomography. PET Clin 2007;2:91–104.
10. Schlemmer HP, Pichler BJ, Schmand M, et al. Simultaneous MR/PET imaging of the human brain: feasibility study. Radiology 2008;248:1028–35.
11. Cho ZH, Son YD, Kim HK, et al. A fusion PET-MRI system with a high-resolution research tomograph-PET and ultra-high field 7.0 T-MRI for the molecular-genetic imaging of the brain. Proteomics 2008;8:1302–23.
12. Knopman DS, DeKosky ST, Cummings JL, et al. Practice parameter: diagnosis of dementia (an evidence-based review). Report of the Quality Standards Subcommittee of the American Academy of Neurology. Neurology 2001;56:1143–53.
13. Devanand DP, Habeck CG, Tabert MH, et al. PET network abnormalities and cognitive decline in patients with mild cognitive impairment. Neuropsychopharmacology 2006;31:1327–34.
14. Jack CR Jr, Petersen RC, Xu YC, et al. Medial temporal atrophy on MRI in normal aging and very mild Alzheimer's disease. Neurology 1997;49:786–94.
15. Sencakova D, Graff-Radford NR, Willis FB, et al. Hippocampal atrophy correlates with clinical features of Alzheimer disease in African Americans. Arch Neurol 2001;58:1593–7.
16. Vermersch P, Leys D, Scheltens P, et al. Visual rating of hippocampal atrophy: correlation with volumetry. J Neurol Neurosurg Psychiatry 1994;57:1015.
17. Wahlund LO, Julin P, Johansson SE, et al. Visual rating and volumetry of the medial temporal lobe on magnetic resonance imaging in dementia: a comparative study. J Neurol Neurosurg Psychiatry 2000;69:630–5.
18. Bresciani L, Rossi R, Testa C, et al. Visual assessment of medial temporal atrophy on MR films in Alzheimer's disease: comparison with volumetry. Aging Clin Exp Res 2005;17:8–13.
19. Burton EJ, Barber R, Mukaetova-Ladinska EB, et al. Medial temporal lobe atrophy on MRI differentiates Alzheimer's disease from dementia with Lewy bodies and vascular cognitive impairment: a prospective study with pathological verification of diagnosis. Brain 2009;132:195–203.
20. Wahlund LO, Almkvist O, Blennow K, et al. Evidence-based evaluation of magnetic resonance imaging as a diagnostic tool in dementia workup. Top Magn Reson Imaging 2005;16:427–37.
21. Baron JC, Chetelat G, Desgranges B, et al. In vivo mapping of gray matter loss with voxel-based morphometry in mild Alzheimer's disease. Neuroimage 2001;14:298–309.
22. Frisoni GB, Testa C, Zorzan A, et al. Detection of grey matter loss in mild Alzheimer's disease with voxel based morphometry. J Neurol Neurosurg Psychiatry 2002;73:657–64.
23. Boxer AL, Rankin KP, Miller BL, et al. Cinguloparietal atrophy distinguishes Alzheimer disease from semantic dementia. Arch Neurol 2003;60:949–56.
24. Ishii K, Kawachi T, Sasaki H, et al. Voxel-based morphometric comparison between early- and late-onset mild Alzheimer's disease and assessment of diagnostic performance of z score images. AJNR Am J Neuroradiol 2005;26:333–40.
25. Whitwell JL, Shiung MM, Przybelski SA, et al. MRI patterns of atrophy associated with progression to AD in amnestic mild cognitive impairment. Neurology 2008;70:512–20.
26. Short RA, Broderick DF, Patton A, et al. Different patterns of magnetic resonance imaging atrophy for frontotemporal lobar degeneration syndromes. Arch Neurol 2005;62:1106–10.
27. Mummery CJ, Patterson K, Price CJ, et al. A voxel-based morphometry study of semantic dementia: relationship between temporal lobe atrophy and semantic memory. Ann Neurol 2000;47:36–45.
28. Rosen HJ, Gorno-Tempini ML, Goldman WP, et al. Patterns of brain atrophy in frontotemporal dementia and semantic dementia. Neurology 2002;58:198–208.
29. CE Krueger, DL Dean, HJ Rosen, et al. Longitudinal rates of lobar atrophy in frontotemporal dementia, semantic dementia, and Alzheimer's disease. Alzheimer Dis Assoc Disord 2010;24:43–8.
30. Pereira JM, Williams GB, Acosta-Cabronero J, et al. Atrophy patterns in histologic vs clinical groupings of frontotemporal lobar degeneration. Neurology 2009;72:1653–60.
31. Middelkoop HA, van der Flier WM, Burton EJ, et al. Dementia with Lewy bodies and AD are not associated with occipital lobe atrophy on MRI. Neurology 2001;57:2117–20.
32. Tam CW, Burton EJ, McKeith IG, et al. Temporal lobe atrophy on MRI in Parkinson disease with dementia: a comparison with Alzheimer disease and dementia with Lewy bodies. Neurology 2005;64:861–5.
33. Whitwell JL, Weigand SD, Shiung MM, et al. Focal atrophy in dementia with Lewy bodies on MRI: a distinct pattern from Alzheimer's disease. Brain 2007;130:708–19.
34. Kenny ER, Burton EJ, O'Brien JT. A volumetric magnetic resonance imaging study of entorhinal cortex volume in dementia with lewy bodies. A

comparison with Alzheimer's disease and Parkinson's disease with and without dementia. Dement Geriatr Cogn Disord 2008;26:218–25.
35. Boxer AL, Geschwind MD, Belfor N, et al. Patterns of brain atrophy that differentiate corticobasal degeneration syndrome from progressive supranuclear palsy. Arch Neurol 2006;63:81–6.
36. Josephs KA, Whitwell JL, Dickson DW, et al. Voxel-based morphometry in autopsy proven PSP and CBD. Neurobiol Aging 2008;29:280–9.
37. Koyama M, Yagishita A, Nakata Y, et al. Imaging of corticobasal degeneration syndrome. Neuroradiology 2007;49:905–12.
38. Varrone A, Asenbaum S, Vander Borght T, et al. EANM procedure guidelines for PET brain imaging using [18F]FDG, version 2. Eur J Nucl Med Mol Imaging 2009;36:2103–10.
39. Waxman AD, Herholz K, Lewis DH, et al. Society of Nuclear Medicine Procedure Guideline for FDG PET brain imaging. Available at: http://interactive.snm.org/index.cfm?PageID=772. Accessed January 30, 2010.
40. Klunk WE, Engler H, Nordberg A, et al. Imaging brain amyloid in Alzheimer's disease with Pittsburgh Compound-B. Ann Neurol 2004;55:306–19.
41. Cohen RM. The application of positron-emitting molecular imaging tracers in Alzheimer's disease. Mol Imaging Biol 2007;9:204–16.
42. Mosconi L, Nacmias B, Sorbi S, et al. Brain metabolic decreases related to the dose of the ApoE e4 allele in Alzheimer's disease. J Neurol Neurosurg Psychiatry 2004;75:370–6.
43. Nihashi T, Yatsuya H, Hayasaka K, et al. Direct comparison study between FDG-PET and IMP-SPECT for diagnosing Alzheimer's disease using 3D-SSP analysis in the same patients. Radiat Med 2007;25:255–62.
44. Del Sole A, Clerici F, Chiti A, et al. Individual cerebral metabolic deficits in Alzheimer's disease and amnestic mild cognitive impairment: an FDG PET study. Eur J Nucl Med Mol Imaging 2008;35:1357–66.
45. Minoshima S, Giordani B, Berent S, et al. Metabolic reduction in the posterior cingulate cortex in very early Alzheimer's disease. Ann Neurol 1997;42:85–94.
46. Silverman DH, Small GW, Chang CY, et al. Positron emission tomography in evaluation of dementia: regional brain metabolism and long-term outcome. JAMA 2001;286:2120–7.
47. Foster NL, Heidebrink JL, Clark CM, et al. FDG-PET improves accuracy in distinguishing frontotemporal dementia and Alzheimer's disease. Brain 2007;130:2616–35.
48. Ishii K, Imamura T, Sasaki M, et al. Regional cerebral glucose metabolism in dementia with Lewy bodies and Alzheimer's disease. Neurology 1998;51:125–30.
49. Kerrouche N, Herholz K, Mielke R, et al. 18FDG PET in vascular dementia: differentiation from Alzheimer's disease using voxel-based multivariate analysis. J Cereb Blood Flow Metab 2006;26:1213–21.
50. Edison P, Archer HA, Hinz R, et al. Amyloid, hypometabolism, and cognition in Alzheimer disease: an [11C]PIB and [18F]FDG PET study. Neurology 2007;68:501–8.
51. Jack CR Jr, Lowe VJ, Senjem ML, et al. 11C PiB and structural MRI provide complementary information in imaging of Alzheimer's disease and amnestic mild cognitive impairment. Brain 2008;131:665–80.
52. Nelissen N, Van Laere K, Thurfjell L, et al. Phase 1 study of the Pittsburgh compound B derivative 18F-flutemetamol in healthy volunteers and patients with probable Alzheimer disease. J Nucl Med 2009;50:1251–9.
53. Engler H, Santillo AF, Wang SX, et al. In vivo amyloid imaging with PET in frontotemporal dementia. Eur J Nucl Med Mol Imaging 2008;35:100–6.
54. Rabinovici GD, Furst AJ, O'Neil JP, et al. 11C-PIB PET imaging in Alzheimer disease and frontotemporal lobar degeneration. Neurology 2007;68:1205–12.
55. Neary D, Snowden JS, Gustafson L, et al. Frontotemporal lobar degeneration: a consensus on clinical diagnostic criteria. Neurology 1998;51:1546–54.
56. Ishii K, Sakamoto S, Sasaki M, et al. Cerebral glucose metabolism in patients with frontotemporal dementia. J Nucl Med 1998;39:1875–8.
57. Jeong Y, Song YM, Chung PW, et al. Correlation of ventricular asymmetry with metabolic asymmetry in frontotemporal dementia. J Neuroradiol 2005;32:247–54.
58. Mirzaei S, Knoll P, Koehn H, et al. Assessment of diffuse Lewy body disease by 2-[18F]fluoro-2-deoxy-D-glucose positron emission tomography (FDG PET). BMC Nucl Med 2003;3:1.
59. Gilman S, Koeppe RA, Little R, et al. Differentiation of Alzheimer's disease from dementia with Lewy bodies utilizing positron emission tomography with [18F]fluorodeoxyglucose and neuropsychological testing. Exp Neurol 2005;191(Suppl 1):S95–103.
60. Ishii K, Soma T, Kono AK, et al. Comparison of regional brain volume and glucose metabolism between patients with mild dementia with lewy bodies and those with mild Alzheimer's disease. J Nucl Med 2007;48:704–11.
61. Okamura N, Arai H, Higuchi M, et al. [18F]FDG-PET study in dementia with Lewy bodies and Alzheimer's disease. Prog Neuropsychopharmacol Biol Psychiatry 2001;25:447–56.

62. Ransmayr G, Seppi K, Donnemiller E, et al. Striatal dopamine transporter function in dementia with Lewy bodies and Parkinson's disease. Eur J Nucl Med 2001;28:1523–8.
63. McKeith I, O'Brien J, Walker Z, et al. Sensitivity and specificity of dopamine transporter imaging with 123I-FP-CIT SPECT in dementia with Lewy bodies: a phase III, multicentre study. Lancet Neurol 2007; 6:305–13.
64. Eckert T, Barnes A, Dhawan V, et al. FDG PET in the differential diagnosis of parkinsonian disorders. Neuroimage 2005;26:912–21.
65. Juh R, Pae CU, Kim TS, et al. Cerebral glucose metabolism in corticobasal degeneration comparison with progressive supranuclear palsy using statistical mapping analysis. Neurosci Lett 2005;383:22–7.
66. Coulier IM, de Vries JJ, Leenders KL. Is FDG-PET a useful tool in clinical practice for diagnosing corticobasal ganglionic degeneration? Mov Disord 2003;18:1175–8.
67. Garraux G, Salmon E, Peigneux P, et al. Voxel-based distribution of metabolic impairment in corticobasal degeneration. Mov Disord 2000;15: 894–904.
68. Chow TW, Binns MA, Freedman M, et al. Overlap in frontotemporal atrophy between normal aging and patients with frontotemporal dementias. Alzheimer Dis Assoc Disord 2008;22:327–35.
69. Alavi A, Newberg AB, Souder E, et al. Quantitative analysis of PET and MRI data in normal aging and Alzheimer's disease: atrophy weighted total brain metabolism and absolute whole brain metabolism as reliable discriminators. J Nucl Med 1993;34: 1681–7.
70. Chawluk J, Alavi A, Dann R, et al. Positron emission tomography in aging and dementia: effect of cerebral atrophy. J Nucl Med 1987;28:431–7.
71. Ibanez V, Pietrini P, Alexander GE, et al. Regional glucose metabolic abnormalities are not the result of atrophy in Alzheimer's disease. Neurology 1998;50:1585–93.
72. Chetelat G, Desgranges B, Landeau B, et al. Direct voxel-based comparison between grey matter hypometabolism and atrophy in Alzheimer's disease. Brain 2008;131:60–71.
73. He Y, Wang L, Zang Y, et al. Regional coherence changes in the early stages of Alzheimer's disease: a combined structural and resting-state functional MRI study. Neuroimage 2007;35:488–500.
74. Morbelli S, Piccardo A, Villavecchia G, et al. Mapping brain morphological and functional conversion patterns in amnestic MCI: a voxel-based MRI and FDG-PET study. Eur J Nucl Med Mol Imaging 2010;37:36–45.
75. Wienhard K, Schmand M, Casey ME, et al. The ECAT HRRT: performance and first clinical application of the new high resolution research tomograph. IEEE Trans Nucl Sci 2002;49:104–10.
76. Karp JS, Surti S, Daube-Witherspoon ME, et al. Performance of a brain PET camera based on anger-logic gadolinium oxyorthosilicate detectors. J Nucl Med 2003;44:1340–9.
77. Watanabe M, Shimizu K, Omura T, et al. A new high-resolution PET scanner dedicated to brain research. IEEE Trans Nucl Sci 2002;49:634–9.
78. Karp JS, Freifelder R, Geagan MJ, et al. Three-dimensional imaging characteristics of the HEAD PENN-PET scanner. J Nucl Med 1997;38:636–43.
79. Yamaya T, Hagiwara N, Obi T, et al. Preliminary resolution performance of the prototype system for a 4-layer DOI-PET scanner: jPET-D4. IEEE Trans Nucl Sci 2006;53:1123–8.
80. K Ziemons, R Achten, E Auffray, et al. The ClearPET™ neuro scanner: a dedicated LSO/LuYAP phoswich small animal PET scanner. In: Seibert JA, editor. IEEE Nuclear Science Symposium Conference Record, vol. 4. Rome (Italy), October 19–22, 2004. p. 2430–3.
81. Braem A, Chamizo Llatas M, Chesi E, et al. Feasibility of a novel design of high-resolution parallax-free Compton enhanced PET scanner dedicated to brain research. Phys Med Biol 2004;49:2547–62.
82. Braem A, Chesi E, Joram C, et al. Wavelength shifter strips and G-APD arrays for the read-out of the z-coordinate in axial PET modules. Nuclear Instruments and Methods in Physics Research Section A 2008;586:300–8.
83. Worstell W, Adler S, Domigan P, et al. Dynamic brain imaging with low injection dose using the NeuroPET [abstract]. J Nucl Med 2009;50:137P.
84. Vaska P, Woody CL, Schlyer DJ, et al. RatCAP: miniaturized head-mounted PET for conscious rodent brain imaging. IEEE Trans Nucl Sci 2004; 51:2718–22.
85. Yamamoto S, Honda M, Shimizu K, et al. Development of PET-Hat: Wearable PET system for brain research [abstract]. J Nucl Med 2009;50:1532.
86. Morimoto Y, Ueno Y, Tsuchiya K, et al. Performance of a prototype brain PET scanner based on semiconductor detectors. J Nucl Med 2008;49:122P [abstract].
87. Trebossen R, Comtat C, Brulon V, et al. Comparison of two commercial whole body PET systems based on LSO and BGO crystals respectively for brain imaging. Med Phys 2009;36:1399–409.
88. van Velden FHP, Kloet RW, van Berckel BNM, et al. HRRT versus HR+ human brain PET studies: an interscanner test-retest study. J Nucl Med 2009; 50:693–702.
89. Woods RP, Mazziotta JC, Cherry SR. MRI-PET registration with automated algorithm. J Comput Assist Tomogr 1993;17:536–46.

90. Pietrzyk U, Herholz K, Fink G, et al. An interactive technique for three-dimensional image registration: validation for PET, SPECT, MRI and CT brain studies. J Nucl Med 1994;35:2011–8.
91. Slomka P, Baum R. Multimodality image registration with software: state-of-the-art. Eur J Nucl Med Mol Imaging 2009;36:44–55.
92. Hammer BE, Christensen NL, Heil BG. Use of a magnetic field to increase the spatial resolution of positron emission tomography. Med Phys 1994; 21:1917–20.
93. Holdsworth SJ, Bammer R. Magnetic resonance imaging techniques: fMRI, DWI, and PWI. Semin Neurol 2008;28:395–406.
94. Talairach J, Tournoux P. Co-planar atlas of the human brain. New York: Thieme Medical Publishers; 1988.
95. Roland PE, Zilles K. Brain atlases—a new research tool. Trends Neurosci 1994;17:458–67.
96. Friston K, Ashburner J, Heather J, et al. Statistical parametric mapping. Available at: http://www.fil.ion.ucl.ac.uk/spm. Accessed February 10, 2010. The Wellcome Department of Cognitive Neurology, University College London. 1999.
97. Minoshima S, Koeppe RA, Frey KA, et al. Stereotactic PET atlas of the human brain: aid for visual interpretation of functional brain images. J Nucl Med 1994;35:949–54.
98. Slomka PJ, Radau P, Hurwitz GA, et al. Automated three-dimensional quantification of myocardial perfusion and brain SPECT. Comput Med Imaging Graph 2001;25:153–64.
99. Herholz K, Salmon E, Perani D, et al. Discrimination between Alzheimer dementia and controls by automated analysis of multicenter FDG PET. Neuroimage 2002;17:302–16.
100. Sanchez-Crespo A, Andreo P, Larsson SA. Positron flight in human tissues and its influence on PET image spatial resolution. Eur J Nucl Med Mol Imaging 2004;31:44–51.
101. Rousset O, Rahmim A, Alavi A, et al. Partial volume correction strategies in PET. PET Clin 2007;2:235–49.
102. Zaidi H, Montandon M-L. Scatter compensation techniques in PET. PET Clin 2007;2:219–34.
103. Zaidi H, Montandon M-L, Meikle S. Strategies for attenuation compensation in neurological PET studies. Neuroimage 2007;34:518–41.
104. Rahmim A, Rousset O, Zaidi H. Strategies for motion tracking and correction in PET. PET Clin 2007;2:251–66.
105. Reader AJ, Zaidi H. Advances in PET image reconstruction. PET Clin 2007;2:173–90.
106. Meltzer CC, Cantwell MN, Greer PJ, et al. Does cerebral blood flow decline in healthy aging? A PET study with partial-volume correction. J Nucl Med 2000;41:1842–8.
107. Muller-Gartner HW, Links JM, Prince JL, et al. Measurement of radiotracer concentration in brain gray matter using positron emission tomography: MRI-based correction for partial volume effects. J Cereb Blood Flow Metab 1992;12:571–83.
108. Matsuda H, Ohnishi T, Asada T, et al. Correction for partial-volume effects on brain perfusion SPECT in healthy men. J Nucl Med 2003;44:1243–52.
109. Meltzer CC, Kinahan PE, Greer PJ, et al. Comparative evaluation of MR-based partial-volume correction schemes for PET. J Nucl Med 1999;40:2053–65.
110. Zaidi H, Ruest T, Schoenahl F, et al. Comparative evaluation of statistical brain MR image segmentation algorithms and their impact on partial volume effect correction in PET. Neuroimage 2006;32: 1591–607.
111. Tohka J, Reilhac A. Deconvolution-based partial volume correction in Raclopride-PET and Monte Carlo comparison to MR-based method. Neuroimage 2008;39:1570–84.
112. Boussion N, Hatt M, Lamare F, et al. A multiresolution image based approach for correction of partial volume effects in emission tomography. Phys Med Biol 2006;51:1857–76.
113. Shidahara M, Tsoumpas C, Hammers A, et al. Functional and structural synergy for resolution recovery and partial volume correction in brain PET. Neuroimage 2009;44:340–8.
114. Baete K, Nuyts J, Laere KV, et al. Evaluation of anatomy based reconstruction for partial volume correction in brain FDG-PET. Neuroimage 2004; 23:305–17.
115. M Montandon, F Assal, O Ratib, et al. MRI-guided voxel-based partial volume effect correction in brain PET: assessment of the impact of 3 MR image segmentation algorithms. 15th Annual Meeting, Organization for Human Brain Mapping (HBM). San Francisco, June 18–23, 2009;47:365.
116. Kohn MI, Tanna NK, Herman GT, et al. Analysis of brain and cerebrospinal fluid volumes with MR imaging. Part I. Methods, reliability, and validation. Radiology 1991;178:115–22.
117. Bural GG, Zhuge Y, Torigian DA, et al. Partial volume correction and segmentation allows accurate measurement of SUV for the grey matter in the brain [abstract]. J Nucl Med 2006;47:9P.
118. Basu S, Zaidi H, Houseni M, et al. Novel quantitative techniques for assessing regional and global function and structure based on modern imaging modalities: implications for normal variation, aging and diseased states. Semin Nucl Med 2007;37: 223–39.
119. Zaidi H, Montandon M, Alavi A. The clinical role of fusion imaging using PET, CT and MRI. Magn Reson Imaging Clin N Am 2010;18:133–49.

Evolving Role of Modern Structural and Functional MR Imaging Techniques for Assessing Neuropsychiatric Disorders

Paolo Nucifora, MD, PhD

KEYWORDS

- Magnetic resonance imaging • Functional MR imaging
- Diffusion tensor imaging • Mental illness

The imaging appearance of neuropsychiatric disorders has evolved dramatically in the past decade, but the reasoning that underlies a modern neuroimaging study is remarkably similar to that of a century ago. To understand mental illness, investigators have typically taken two approaches. The lesion-based approach seeks to localize a specific structural abnormality, whereas the behavior-based approach seeks to characterize the activity and interaction of abnormal networks. These parallel lines of thought lead from the historical work of Broca and Kraepelin directly to the functional and structural paradigms used to evaluate the brain today, and they are likely to inform future studies using PET, MRI, or multimodal approaches.

MORPHOMETRIC MR IMAGING

The evolution of MR imaging in assessing neuropsychiatric disorders has resulted from the synergy between rapid advances in two distinct fields: signal acquisition and image processing. With the development of high-field strength scanners and modern parallel acquisition techniques, signal-to-noise ratios in routine imaging have improved sufficiently to resolve submillimeter features of the brain. Whole brain volumes as well as tissue volumes—gray matter, white matter, and cerebrospinal fluid—can readily be determined. However, neuroanatomists have known for more than a century that the effect of a lesion in the brain depends as much on its location as on the tissue involved. Thus, a high-resolution image of the brain cannot be evaluated fully without some sort of map, linking its features to a standard reference. Previously the domain of an experienced neuroanatomist, this task has increasingly been performed with automated registration, also known as spatial normalization. A sophisticated algorithm is required to find regions of the brain that correspond accurately to each other in different individuals, but the exponential growth of computing power has made automated registration widely available.[1] Today it is possible to scan a patient and promptly link every voxel in the brain to its counterpart in a brain atlas. This allows investigators to evaluate a cohort of patients for consistent abnormalities involving only a few millimeters of tissue, which would be a difficult task by visual inspection even for an experienced neuroradiologist. In addition, the cortical surface can be rearranged to account for its topology, so that two cortical voxels in close

Department of Radiology, University of Pennsylvania, 3400 Spruce Street, Philadelphia, PA 19104, USA
E-mail address: paolo.nucifora@uphs.upenn.edu

PET Clin 5 (2010) 169–183
doi:10.1016/j.cpet.2010.03.004

apposition across a sulcus are treated differently from two cortical voxels in the same gyrus.[2] This permits a precise estimate of cortical thickness, which can only be crudely estimated by visual inspection but may be more biologically relevant than tissue volume.

FUNCTIONAL MR IMAGING

Similar advances in MR imaging acquisition and postprocessing have driven the evolution of functional MR imaging (fMR imaging). Its most common implementation is through blood oxygen-level dependent–(BOLD) fMR imaging, which relies on signal changes that typically accompany neural activity and are caused by increases in local hemoglobin saturation.[3] The degree of signal change is too small to detect by visual inspection, so activation during a BOLD-fMR imaging experiment is localized through a statistical analysis of all brain voxels over multiple time points. To establish statistical power, a large number of images are acquired at short time intervals, which in turn requires sacrificing spatial resolution. The output of a BOLD-fMR imaging experiment is typically a map of all voxels whose signal demonstrates a significant correlation with a particular stimulus or behavior. In addition, the architecture of neural networks can be investigated using a functional connectivity analysis, which produces a map of all voxels whose signal is significantly correlated to the signal of other voxels.[4] Voxels showing functional connectivity at rest are thought to form the "default mode network" that has also been observed using PET.[5] Because definitions of mental illness generally involve behavioral observations and theories of mental illness are frequently based on cognitive networks, fMR imaging has understandably been embraced by neuropsychiatrists investigating an organic basis for disease.

DIFFUSION TENSOR IMAGING

Whereas fMR imaging is used mainly in gray matter, diffusion tensor imaging (DTI) is used mainly to evaluate white matter. The development of DTI has been driven by improvements in MR imaging scanner gradients, which are rapidly reconfigurable magnetic fields that are superimposed on a powerful constant magnetic field to produce spatial order during MR image acquisition. Introducing opposing gradient pairs, known as motion-probing gradients, reduces the signal of any voxel that contains water molecules moving parallel to the gradients.[6] Although any type of water motion will have an effect, diffusion-weighting in brain tissue is achieved if the predominant mode of motion on the time scale of the scan is by self-diffusion. Typically, this requires a rapid scan that sacrifices spatial resolution. If the scan is repeated with motion-probing gradients applied in different orientations, a model of water diffusion can be obtained for every voxel. In the ventricles, for example, diffusion is observed to occur equally in all directions. In other regions, diffusion may demonstrate a directional preference known as diffusion anisotropy. This is the theoretical basis for DTI.

Empirically, it has been shown that white matter demonstrates strong diffusion anisotropy, and diffusion occurs preferentially in directions parallel to axon bundles. Fractional anisotropy (FA), a metric for the degree of diffusion anisotropy, has been correlated to microstructural integrity in voxels containing white matter. Presumably, water movement is affected by the parallel organization of intact microstructural features of white matter, including myelin sheaths, plasma membranes, and cytoskeletal elements. Automated registration of DTI data presents specific challenges due to their multidimensional nature. One of the more popular approaches, tract-based spatial statistics (TBSS), uses a skeletal model of white matter to align white matter tracts.[7] More detailed representations of white matter connectivity can be produced using diffusion tractography, which traces water diffusion voxel-by-voxel to generate a three-dimensional rendering of white matter fibers.[4,8,9] Quantification of tractography results has not yet been standardized and may require the use of full-tensor registration.[10,11] Although DTI is not a functional imaging modality, its measurements of white matter connectivity often complement functional observations. Increasingly, it is used as a bridge between structural and functional approaches.

All of these MR imaging techniques have been used in the study of neuropsychiatric disorders. In the remainder of this article, the use of MR imaging will be illustrated in specific clinical settings.

AUTISM SPECTRUM DISORDER

The diagnosis of autism spectrum disorder (ASD) comprises autism as well as Asperger syndrome and pervasive developmental disorder, which share features such as impaired social interaction. Several studies have correlated neuropsychologic test performance and clinical variables for ASD with regional brain volumes.[12,13] More strikingly, patients with ASD have repeatedly shown increased global cerebral volumes, particularly early in life.[14] Although the corpus callosum is generally found to be smaller in patients with autism, some studies have suggested that subcortical white matter may be overabundant.[15,16] For example, among intellectually disabled children who had globally decreased brain volume, the subgroup with ASD nevertheless demonstrated increased white matter volumes in the superior temporal gyrus.[17] A recent closer inspection of boys with ASD demonstrated increased brain volumes that were most apparent in the frontal lobes, as well as a more widespread pattern of white matter excess accompanied by gray matter deficiency, whereas another study demonstrated increased gray matter volume in the left frontal and temporal lobes.[18,19] The role of the cerebellum in ASD is less clear, and conflicting results have been reported regarding cerebellar volumes.[13,19–22]

These findings run counter with the natural instinct to equate brain pathology with tissue loss, but they should be seen in the context of preadolescent brain development. Neurons mature by pruning unnecessary connections, and abnormal development could feasibly be manifested as increased volume at an early age. Functional connectivity studies using BOLD-fMR imaging provide additional evidence for abnormal connectivity in ASD. A recent study demonstrated decreased functional connectivity between the right superior frontal gyrus and the posterior cingulate cortex in patients with ASD at rest.[23] Small areas in the right temporal lobe and right parahippocampal gyrus demonstrated stronger connectivity. The degree of functional connectivity in these regions was correlated with behavioral and social variables. Another study demonstrated decreased functional correlation bilaterally between the inferior parietal lobule and the inferior frontal gyrus in patients with ASD performing a verbal fluency task.[24] A meta-analysis of ASD across multiple functional modalities found decreased activation in the posterior cingulate cortex as well as the anterior cingulate cortex during social tasks, but increased activation in the anterior cingulate cortex and the supplemental motor area during nonsocial tasks (**Fig. 1**).[25]

DTI of patients with ASD can offer insight into both volumetric and functional MR imaging findings. For example, decreased FA in ASD has been demonstrated in medial frontal subcortical white matter (**Fig. 2**), which is consistent with findings of abnormal activation in prefrontal cortex.[26] Both BOLD-fMR imaging and DTI measures were correlated with a clinical index of restricted and repetitive behavior. Other

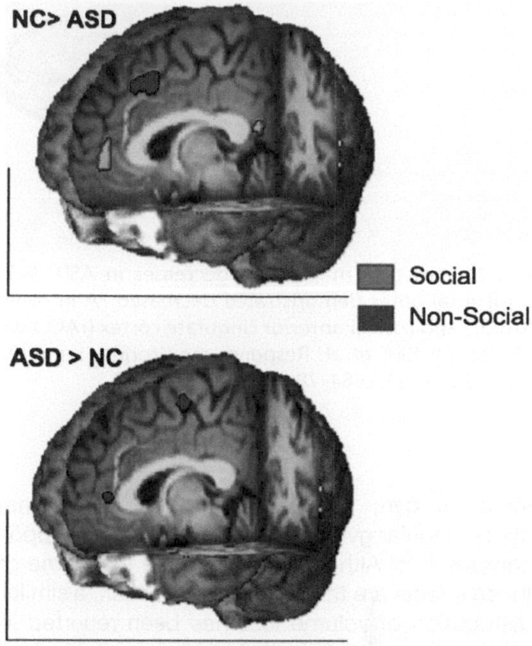

Fig. 1. Results of meta-analysis of functional studies of ASD during social and nonsocial tasks. Compared with controls (NC), patients with ASD demonstrated decreased activation in anterior cingulate cortex and posterior cingulate cortex during social tasks as well as decreased activation in the presupplementary motor area during nonsocial tasks. However, they demonstrated increased activation in anterior cingulate cortex and supplementary motor area during nonsocial tasks. (*Adapted from* Di Martino A, Ross K, Uddin LQ, et al. Functional brain correlates of social and nonsocial processes in autism spectrum disorders: an activation likelihood estimation meta-analysis. Biol Psychiatry 2009;65:63–74; with permission.)

studies have shown abnormal FA in the corpus callosum and a relationship between callosal FA and IQ in adolescents with ASD.[15] In keeping with the volumetric distinctions between early age and adulthood, Ben Bashat and colleagues[27] reported increased white matter FA in young children with ASD.

SCHIZOPHRENIA

Schizophrenia is a cognitive disorder usually beginning in adolescence. It is manifested by "negative symptoms" including social withdrawal and diminished affect, and "positive symptoms" including psychotic features. An association between chronic schizophrenia and decreased cerebral volume is fairly well established.[28,29] Focal regions of volume loss or heterogeneity have been described in orbitofrontal cortex; superior and inferior frontal gyri; superior, inferior, and middle

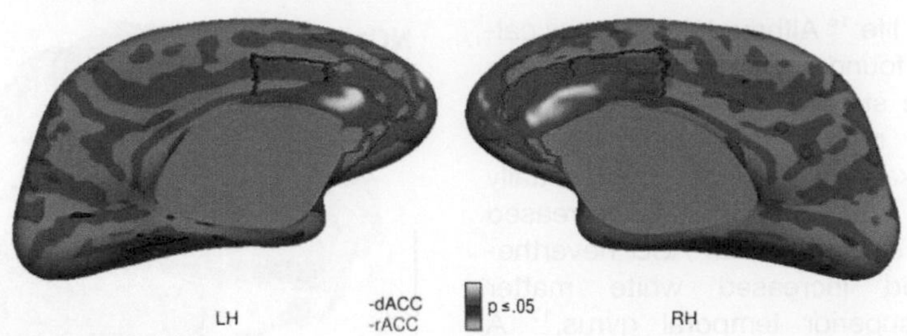

Fig. 2. Statistical map of FA decreases in ASD. Subcortical white matter in left (LH) and right (RH) medial prefrontal areas demonstrated decreased FA in comparison with controls. The dorsal anterior cingulate cortex (dACC) and rostral anterior cingulate cortex (rACC) were outlined for reference. (*Adapted from* Thakkar KN, Polli FE, Joseph RM, et al. Response monitoring, repetitive behaviour and anterior cingulate abnormalities in ASD. Brain 2008;131:2464–78; with permission.)

temporal gyri; cingulate cortex, supramarginal gyrus, angular gyrus, lingual gyrus, and the hippocampus.[30–33] Although it is possible that some of these effects are the result of medication, a similar distribution of volume loss has been reported in patients presenting in their first episode, before substantial medical treatment.[34,35]

The most consistent DTI findings in schizophrenia are reductions in microstructural integrity of frontal and temporal white matter.[36,37] Decreased FA has also been reported in the parietal lobes and cerebellum.[38,39] A wide variety of white matter tracts have been implicated in schizophrenia using diffusion tractography, including the uncinate fasciculus and thalamocortical projections.[36,37,40–42] The arcuate fasciculus has demonstrated mixed findings,[43,44] but reports of increased connectivity in this language-associated tract have suggested a role in the auditory hallucinations frequently manifested in schizophrenia.

Patients experiencing auditory hallucinations during BOLD-fMR imaging have demonstrated activation of primary auditory cortex that is similar to that observed when hearing external speech.[45] This pattern is not observed during a normal inner dialog in a healthy person, indicating a fundamental difference in the neural processing of hallucinations (**Fig. 3**). Negative symptoms have also been investigated with functional imaging. For example, the severity of affect flattening in schizophrenia has been correlated to the degree of BOLD signal change in the amygdala during the successful identification of fearful facial expressions.[46] In this task, patients with schizophrenia demonstrated decreased activation of the amygdala and other limbic structures. Both negative and positive symptoms have been found to correlate to the degree of functional connectivity in medial frontal and anterior cingulate cortex.[47] In addition, regions of altered functional connectivity were found to overlap with regions of altered white matter microstructure. In other studies, abnormal connectivity has been demonstrated in individuals at very early stages of disease and even those at risk of psychosis without a diagnosis of schizophrenia.[48,49] Together, these findings suggest that cerebral disconnectivity may play an important role in schizophrenia, and they complement PET findings of abnormalities in cerebral function as well as in dopaminergic and serotonergic systems.

OBSESSIVE-COMPULSIVE DISORDER

Obsessive-compulsive disorder (OCD) is a common anxiety disorder characterized by intrusive thoughts and repetitive behaviors, often with the awareness that they are irrational. Two recent meta-analyses found increased volumes in the lenticular nucleus and thalamus with direct correlations between symptom severity and tissue volume.[50,51] Decreased volumes were found in anterior cingulate cortex and orbitofrontal cortex. Using voxel-based morphometry, a correlation has been demonstrated between symptom severity and white matter volumes in the anterior limb of the internal capsule bilaterally, although as a group the OCD patients did not differ significantly from healthy controls.[52]

Mixed volumetric findings in OCD are parallel to DTI observations of white matter microstructure, with findings of increased and decreased FA in different regions of white matter. Foci of increased FA have been reported in the cingulum, corpus callosum, centrum semiovale, subinsular white matter, medial frontal white matter, internal capsule, corpus callosum, and lenticular nucleus, which in some cases could no longer be detected after treatment.[53–56] In other studies of OCD, the cingulum and corpus callosum demonstrated foci

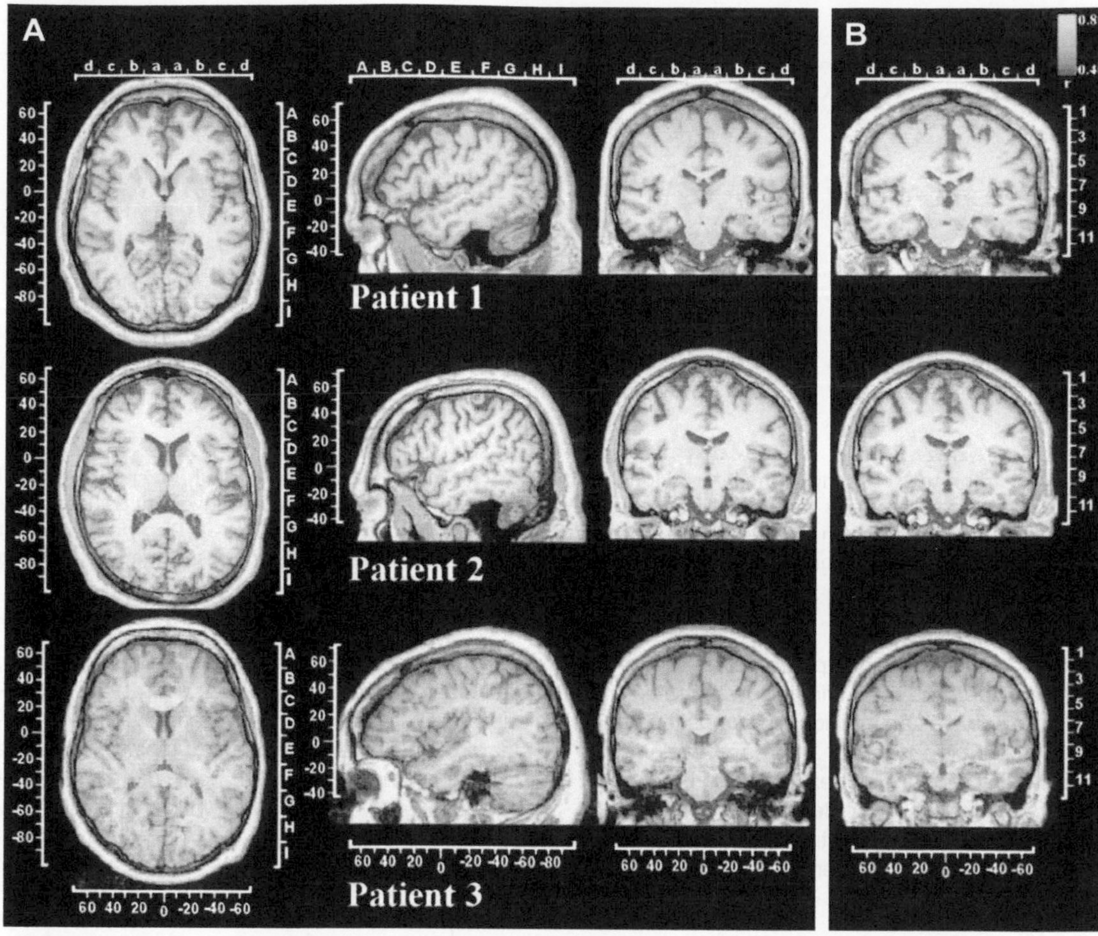

Fig. 3. Activation during auditory hallucinations in schizophrenia resembled activation during normal speech reception. BOLD-fMR imaging maps for three patients with schizophrenia during self-reported auditory hallucinations (*A*) and binaural speech reception (*B*). In both cases, primary auditory cortex was activated. (*Adapted from* Dierks T, Linden DE, Jandl M, et al. Activation of Heschl's gyrus during auditory hallucinations. Neuron 1999;22:615–21; with permission.)

of decreased FA, as have the inferior fronto-occipital fasciculus and regions of inferior parietal white matter (**Fig. 4**).[55,57,58]

Patients with OCD have also demonstrated mixed changes in functional connectivity, as measured by BOLD-fMR imaging. A recent study of OCD by Harrison and colleagues[59] showed greater functional connectivity of orbitofrontal cortex with the nucleus accumbens and the ventral putamen. In this study, connectivity between orbitofrontal cortex and the ventral striatum was strongly correlated with symptom severity scores (**Fig. 5**). However, decreased connectivity was found between orbitofrontal cortex and the dorsal putamen. In other studies, decreased BOLD signal was demonstrated in orbitofrontal cortex, the inferior frontal gyrus, and the medial frontal gyrus during inhibition tasks and in orbitofrontal cortex during a learning task.[60–62] The diverse manifestations of OCD were explored by An and colleagues,[63] who grouped patients with hoarding behavior separately from those without the behavior. They found that the former group showed increased activation in ventromedial prefrontal cortex when asked to imagine discarding objects that are frequently hoarded. The degree of activation was directly correlated to the level of anxiety reported by these patients.

MAJOR DEPRESSIVE DISORDER

Major depressive disorder (MDD) is a common mood disorder characterized by recurrent depressive episodes. Chen and colleagues[64] found that the volume of the anterior cingulate cortex was

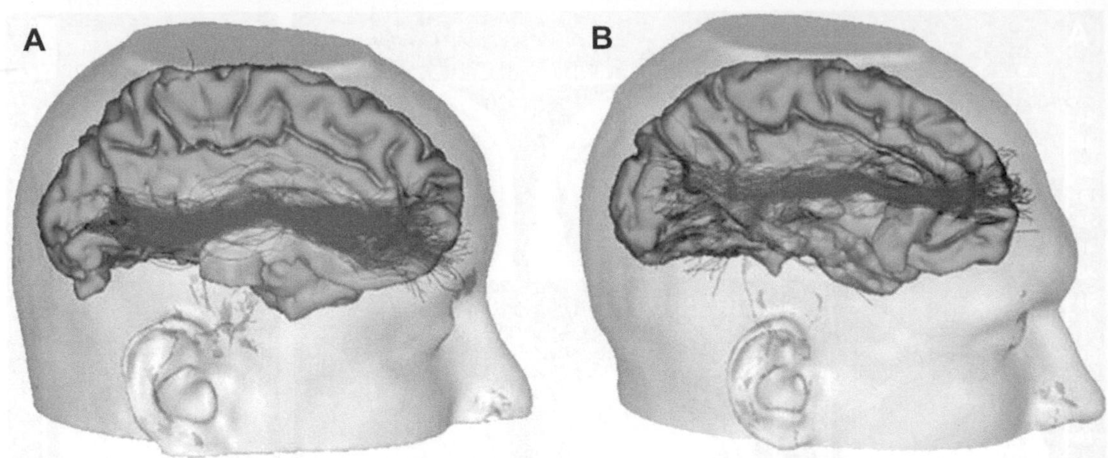

Fig. 4. Diffusion tractography of the inferior longitudinal fasciculus in OCD. As compared with a healthy control (*A*), the posterior segments of the inferior longitudinal fasciculus demonstrate qualitatively decreased fiber coherence in a patient with OCD (*B*). (*Adapted from* Garibotto V, Scifo P, Gorini A, et al. Disorganization of anatomical connectivity in obsessive compulsive disorder: a multi-parameter diffusion tensor imaging study in a subpopulation of patients. Neurobiol Dis 2010;37:468–76; with permission.)

directly correlated with improvement after antidepressant therapy. This finding was sufficiently robust to serve as an individual prognostic for their study population (**Fig. 6**). Decreased volumes in the anterior cingulate cortex have also been noted in boys with subclinical depressive symptoms.[65] More commonly, volumetric studies of patients with depression have demonstrated decreased gray matter volume in the hippocampus bilaterally, especially in the posterior aspect of the hippocampus.[66–68] Loss of gray matter volume appeared to be asymmetric, and typically was more prominent throughout the right cerebral hemisphere (**Fig. 7**).[67] Individuals with a family history

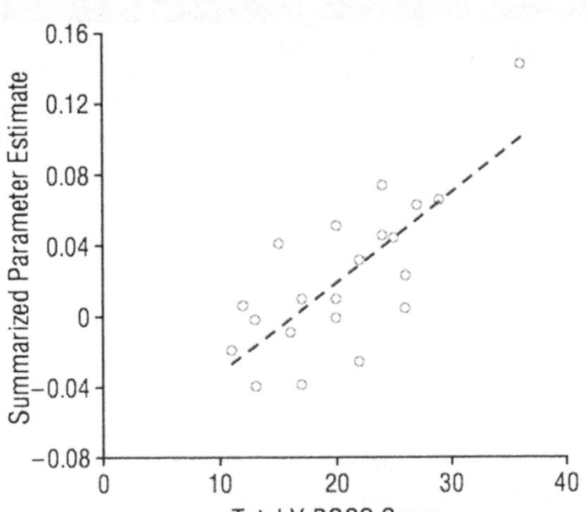

Fig. 5. Correlation between functional connectivity in OCD and symptom severity. An estimate of functional connectivity between orbitofrontal cortex and ventral striatum was plotted against Yale-Brown Obsessive Compulsive Scale (Y-BOCS) severity scores, demonstrating a strong positive correlation. (*Adapted from* Harrison BJ, Soriano-Mas C, Pujol J, et al. Altered corticostriatal functional connectivity in obsessive-compulsive disorder. Arch Gen Psychiatry 2009;66:1189–200; with permission.)

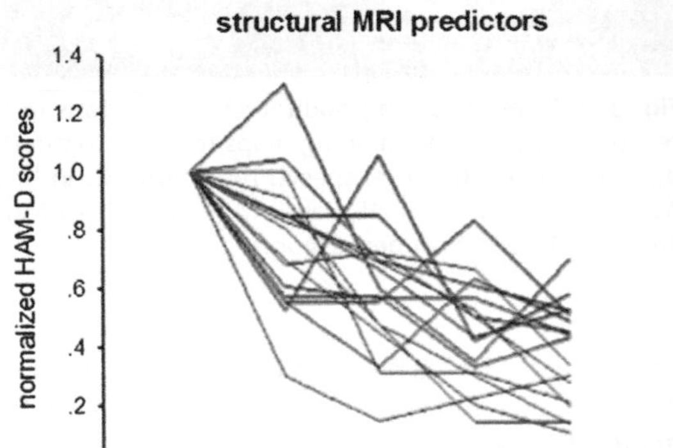

Fig. 6. Structural MR imaging and treatment response to antidepressants. Morphometric MR imaging was used to measure volumes of anterior cingulate cortex, right temporoparietal cortex, and insular cortex of unmedicated patients with MDD. Symptom scores were monitored during treatment for 8 weeks. The line color denotes whether gray matter volumes were above (*red*) or below (*black*) the group median. Patients with greater volumes uniformly improved faster. (*Adapted from* Chen CH, Ridler K, Suckling J, et al. Brain imaging correlates of depressive symptom severity and predictors of symptom improvement after antidepressant treatment. Biol Psychiatry 2007;62:407–14; with permission.)

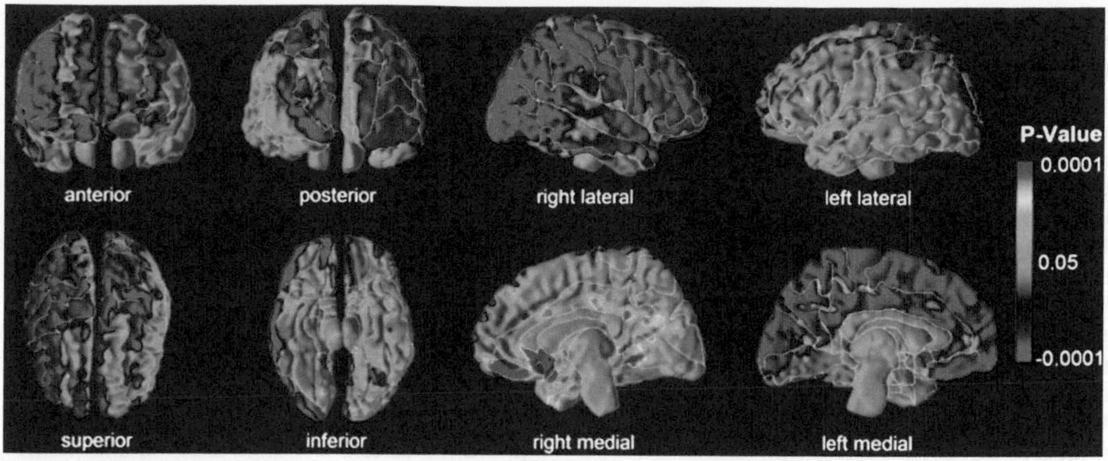

Fig. 7. Surface rendered map of cortical thickness in MDD. Regions of decreased cortical thickness were labeled with cool colors, whereas regions of increased cortical thickness were labeled in warm colors. Patients with MDD demonstrated asymmetric cortical thinning in the medial left hemisphere and lateral right hemisphere. Significance was set at a threshold of $P<.05$ (uncorrected for multiple comparisons). (*Adapted from* Peterson BS, Warner V, Bansal R, et al. Cortical thinning in persons at increased familial risk for major depression. Proc Natl Acad Sci U S A 2009;106:6273–8; with permission.)

of depression, who face a higher risk of anxiety and major depressive disorder, also demonstrated decreased cortical thickness in the right hemisphere.[69] This suggests that cortical asymmetry may precede development of neuropsychiatric symptoms. These findings are similar to PET findings of abnormalities in cortical areas, particular the frontal lobes.

Studies using DTI to evaluate white matter microstructure in MDD have demonstrated areas of reduced FA in prefrontal, parietal, and temporal white matter.[70,71] Symptom severity was found to be inversely related to FA in the anterior limb of the internal capsule.[71] However, other studies found that patients with MDD failed to show any significant differences in FA.[72,73] Abnormalities in white matter microstructure were even more pronounced in geriatric depression. Even after accounting for the effect of age, decreased FA was found in prefrontal, medial temporal, parietal, and occipital white matter.[74–77]

Studies of functional connectivity in MDD have demonstrated mixed findings. Frodl and colleagues[78] showed decreased functional connectivity between orbitofrontal cortex and several medial cortical structures during emotional tasks in patients with MDD. Likewise, Bluhm and colleagues[79] showed decreased functional connectivity between the posterior cingulate cortex and the caudate at rest. However, others have suggested increased functional connectivity to the anterior cingulate from medial cortical structures at rest or during executive processing.[80,81] Patients with MDD have also demonstrated increased task-related activity in the dorsolateral prefrontal cortex during emotion processing.[82] The degree of hyperactivation was found to be correlated with symptom severity.

BIPOLAR DISORDER

Bipolar disorder (BPD) is a mood disorder characterized by manic episodes that may alternate with periods of depression. A sophisticated study of cortical topology produced evidence of abnormal sulcation in BPD.[83] Increased pituitary volumes have been reported, implicating systemic neuroendocrine involvement.[84] In the amygdala, there are conflicting volume measurements that perhaps are due to the confounding effects of medication.[85] In general, volumetric MR imaging studies of patients with BPD tend to report decreased cerebral volumes or increased ventricular volumes, possibly reversed after treatment with mood stabilizers.[86–88]

The most common finding in BPD may be an increased number of T2-hyperintense lesions in the deep or subcortical white matter. This is a fairly nonspecific finding that can be seen in normal aging, but recent studies of BPD continue to demonstrate lesion load that is out of proportion to age.[87,89] A recent meta-analysis of tissue volumetry in BPD confirmed a reduction in white matter volumes.[90] There are conflicting reports regarding the DTI appearance of white matter of patients with BPD, which ultimately may be due to the heterogeneity in medication status. Areas of white matter hyperintensity have demonstrated increased mean diffusivity (MD), possibly related to white matter pathology.[91] Although decreased FA or increased MD have been reported in several regions of white matter, more recent studies have shown increased FA in regions of prefrontal white matter.[91–95] In one study, DTI was used to perform tractography on the white matter pathways connecting the subgenual cingulate cortex to the amygdala and hippocampus, which mainly consist of fibers in the uncinate fasciculus. Increased fiber density was found on the left side, possibly resulting in asymmetric frontotemporal connectivity.[96] Similarly, multiple studies using TBSS have demonstrated increased FA in tracts coursing through medial prefrontal cortex (**Fig. 8**).[97,98]

In a recent study by Wang and colleagues,[99] patients with BPD showed decreased FA in areas thought to subserve connectivity between the pregenual anterior cingulate cortex and the amygdala. Furthermore, reductions in FA were correlated to decreased functional connectivity between these regions, as determined by BOLD-fMR imaging. However, Almeida and colleagues[100] suggested that effective connectivity at rest between the right subgenual cingulate cortex and the right parahippocampal gyrus is increased in BPD. Several other studies have provided evidence of abnormal frontal BOLD-fMR imaging signal during emotion processing or memory tasks. When rating hostility, children with bipolar disorder showed increased limbic activation, mainly in the left amygdala, nucleus accumbens, putamen, and ventrolateral prefrontal cortex.[101] During learning and memory tasks, patients with bipolar disorder have demonstrated abnormal activation of prefrontal cortex, occipital cortex, and the amygdala.[102–104]

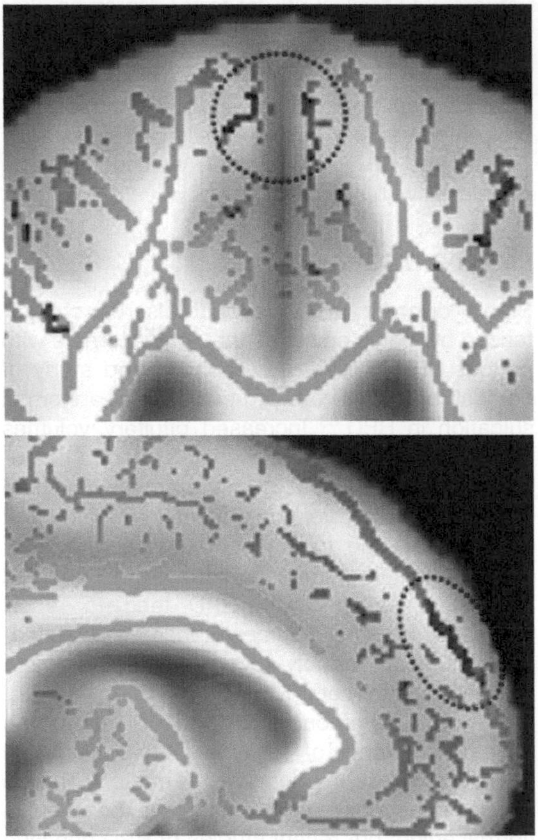

Fig. 8. Regions of abnormal FA in BPD. White matter skeleton (*green*) produced by TBSS demonstrated two clusters of increased FA (*blue*) in patients with BPD, located in medial prefrontal and precentral white matter. (*Adapted from* Wessa M, Houenou J, Leboyer M, et al. Microstructural white matter changes in euthymic bipolar patients: a whole-brain diffusion tensor imaging study. Bipolar Disord 2009;11:504–14; with permission.)

FUTURE DIRECTIONS: IMAGE-DRIVEN GENETICS

The structural and functional MR imaging findings discussed above are just a sample of a large and rapidly evolving body of literature. Complementary PET findings regarding neurotransmitter systems in psychiatric disorders may contribute to a better depiction of their underlying pathophysiology. Several additional trends in neuroimaging are likely to shape future investigations.

Our basic understanding of neuropsychiatric disorders increasingly is underpinned by a convergence of imaging and genetics. New heritable biomarkers of disease susceptibility, known as endophenotypes, are continually being discovered using neuroimaging.

In ASD, which has a fairly well-established pattern of heritability, patients and their unaffected siblings showed similar volume reductions in the amygdala and abnormal activation in the fusiform gyrus during facial recognition.[105] Likewise, young boys with ASD and their asymptomatic fathers demonstrated diminished activity in the right fusiform gyrus when inferring emotional states.[106]

Investigations of the genetics of schizophrenia have focused on several genetic loci with alleles that are associated with increased vulnerability, including dystrobrevin-binding protein 1, catechol-O-methyltransferase, and glutamate decarboxylase 1. These genes, in turn, may lead to new imaging endophenotypes. For example, asymptomatic individuals with susceptibility alleles for the dystrobrevin-binding protein 1and catechol-O-methyltransferase genes have demonstrated areas of reduced cortical volume.[107–109] In contrast, both susceptibility genes have been associated with

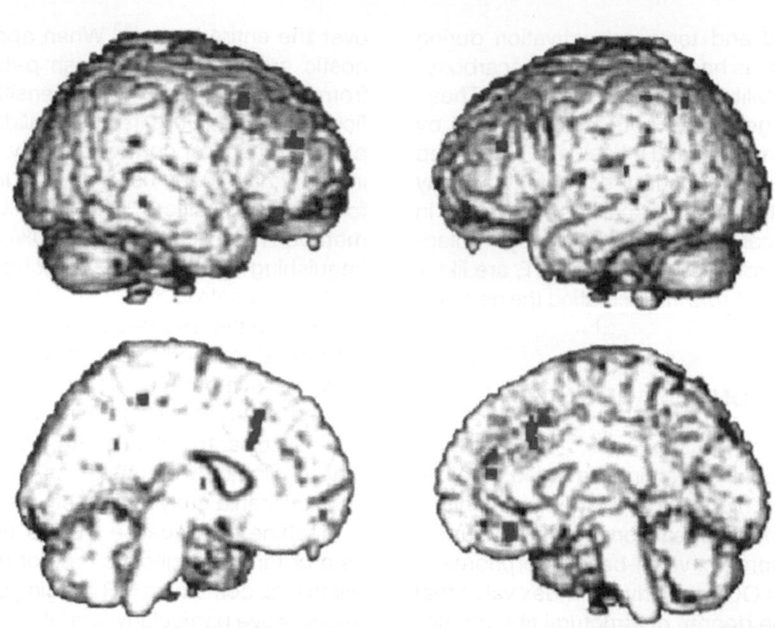

Fig. 9. The effects of catechol-O-methyltransferase genotype on activation during a memory task. Areas in red showed an association between catechol-O-methyltransferase genotype and activation on BOLD-fMR imaging. The Val/Val genotype, considered a risk factor for schizophrenia, was associated with greater activation in these areas than the Met/Met genotype. Individuals with the Val/Met genotype demonstrated intermediate activation. (*Adapted from* Egan MF, Goldberg TE, Kolachana BS, et al. Effect of COMT Val108/158 Met genotype on frontal lobe function and risk for schizophrenia. Proc Natl Acad Sci U S A 2001;98:6917–22; with permission.)

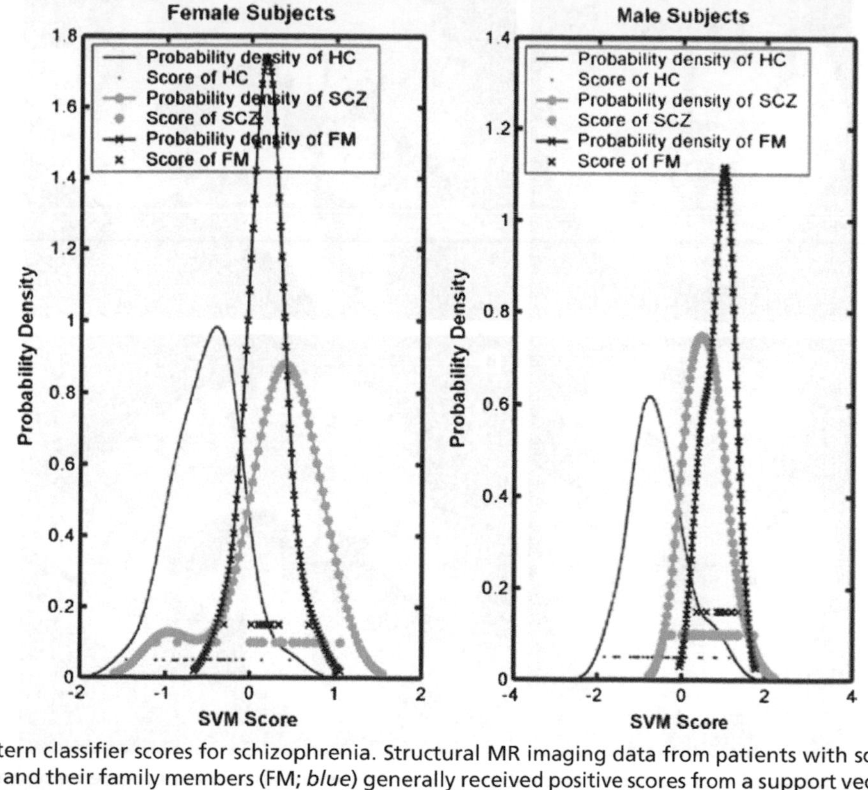

Fig. 10. Pattern classifier scores for schizophrenia. Structural MR imaging data from patients with schizophrenia (SCZ; *green*) and their family members (FM; *blue*) generally received positive scores from a support vector machine (SVM) pattern classifier. MR imaging data from healthy controls (HC; *red*) generally received negative scores. (*Adapted from* Fan Y, Gur RE, Gur RC, et al. Unaffected family members and schizophrenia patients share brain structure patterns: a high-dimensional pattern classification study. Biol Psychiatry 2008;63:118–24; with permission.)

increased frontal and temporal activation during a variety of tasks, as has the glutamate decarboxylase 1 susceptibility allele (**Fig 9**).[110–112] These increases are generally not accompanied by improved performance, and it has been suggested that the genetic component of schizophrenia may involve organizational abnormalities that result in decreased cortical processing efficiency. Molecular imaging approaches, including PET, are likely to play an important role in elucidating the genetics of schizophrenia.

FUTURE DIRECTIONS: IMAGE-BASED DIAGNOSIS

Advances in machine learning have led to algorithms capable of higher-order pattern recognition in images that would appear nonspecific to a human observer. For example, voxel-based morphometry has been used in OCD to derive an index value that encapsulates the degree of structural abnormality over the entire brain.[113] When applied as a diagnostic criterion to distinguish patients with OCD from healthy controls, both sensitivity and specificity exceeded 90% in cross-validation. In schizophrenia, maps of cortical atrophy or white matter integrity have been used to produce learning sets for pattern classifiers. With cross-validation, these methods have achieved over 80% accuracy in distinguishing patients with schizophrenia from healthy controls.[31,114,115] Machine learning methods have also been used to classify patients with predominantly psychotic, disorganized, or negative symptoms.[116] Remarkably, asymptomatic family members of patients have demonstrated scores similar to patients (**Fig. 10**), which suggests that the link between genetics and morphology in schizophrenia may ultimately be discovered by a machine.[117] Because PET is under evaluation as a potential diagnostic tool for neuropsychiatric disorders, combining MR imaging and PET findings might prove particularly fruitful.

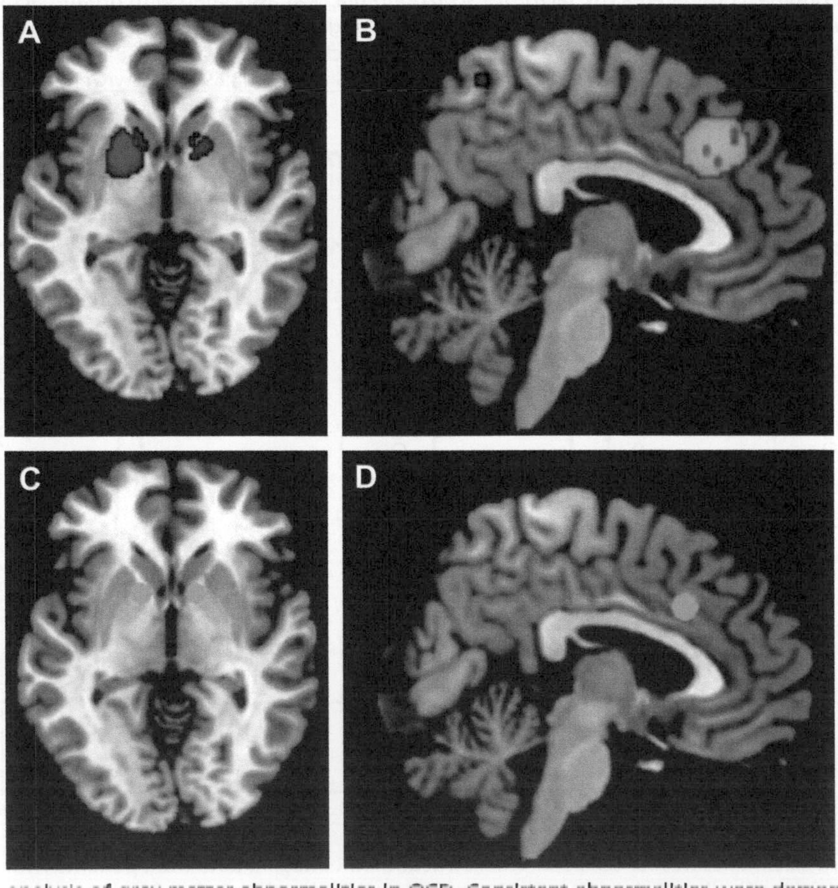

Fig. 11. Meta-analysis of gray matter abnormalities in OCD. Consistent abnormalities were demonstrated in the lenticular nuclei (*A*) and the anterior cingulate (*B*). These regions correspond to typical neurosurgical targets in OCD (*C, D*). (*Adapted from* Radua J, Mataix-Cols D. Voxel-wise meta-analysis of grey matter changes in obsessive-compulsive disorder. Br J Psychiatry 2009;195:393–402; with permission.)

FUTURE DIRECTIONS: IMAGE-GUIDED INTERVENTION

The treatment of OCD and MDD has been transformed by demonstrations of the effectiveness of cingulotomy, capsulotomy, and implantable electrodes in deep brain nuclei.[118–120] In turn, this has sparked an image-guided search for new neurosurgical targets. In OCD, effective interventional targets and imaging abnormalities in the anterior cingulate cortex and internal capsule demonstrate a startling correspondence (**Fig. 11**).[51]

In contrast, effective neurosurgical targets in MDD do not correlate as consistently to focal neuroimaging findings. This may reflect the interaction between focal abnormalities and the widely distributed networks to which they belong. In this context, Gutman and colleagues[121] used tractography to evaluate white matter targets for deep brain stimulation in MDD. They found evidence of widespread connectivity to distant areas of the brain, including some of the areas implicated in MDD.[121] For neurosurgical intervention to be effectively integrated into the treatment of other mental illnesses, additional research will be needed into the mechanisms by which stimulators and directed lesions exert their effects.

SUMMARY

MR imaging has contributed a wealth of knowledge regarding the interaction between structures of the brain and manifestations of neuropsychiatric disorders. Nevertheless, this knowledge has not produced a satisfying answer to the most fundamental question: where does mental illness come from? Unlike neurologists who can localize a weakness to capsular infarction or neurosurgeons who can localize unresponsiveness to a ruptured aneurysm, neuropsychiatrists are still at a loss to explain the origin of the symptoms which they must treat. Functional and structural imaging studies have played a major role in the rapid expansion of knowledge regarding these disorders. However, neuropsychiatry is a long way from becoming a mature science. We are still in the childhood of our endeavor to understand the brain.

REFERENCES

1. Davatzikos C. Voxel-based morphometric analysis using shape transformations. Int Rev Neurobiol 2005;66:125–46.
2. Van Essen DC. Surface-based approaches to spatial localization and registration in primate cerebral cortex. Neuroimage 2004;23(Suppl 1):S97–107.
3. Logothetis NK. What we can do and what we cannot do with fMRI. Nature 2008;453:869–78.
4. Ramnani N, Behrens TE, Penny W, et al. New approaches for exploring anatomical and functional connectivity in the human brain. Biol Psychiatry 2004;56:613–9.
5. Buckner RL, Andrews-Hanna JR, Schacter DL. The brain's default network: anatomy, function, and relevance to disease. Ann N Y Acad Sci 2008;1124:1–38.
6. Le Bihan D, Mangin JF, Poupon C, et al. Diffusion tensor imaging: concepts and applications. J Magn Reson Imaging 2001;13:534–46.
7. Smith SM, Jenkinson M, Johansen-Berg H, et al. Tract-based spatial statistics: voxelwise analysis of multi-subject diffusion data. Neuroimage 2006; 31:1487–505.
8. Conturo TE, Lori NF, Cull TS, et al. Tracking neuronal fiber pathways in the living human brain. Proc Natl Acad Sci U S A 1999;96:10422–7.
9. Mori S, van Zijl PC. Fiber tracking: principles and strategies—a technical review. NMR Biomed 2002;15:468–80.
10. Verma R, Mori S, Shen D, et al. Spatiotemporal maturation patterns of murine brain quantified by diffusion tensor MRI and deformation-based morphometry. Proc Natl Acad Sci U S A 2005; 102:6978–83.
11. Nucifora PG, Verma R, Lee SK, et al. Diffusion-tensor MR imaging and tractography: exploring brain microstructure and connectivity. Radiology 2007;245:367–84.
12. Schumann CM, Barnes CC, Lord C, et al. Amygdala enlargement in toddlers with autism related to severity of social and communication impairments. Biol Psychiatry 2009;66:942–9.
13. Webb SJ, Sparks BF, Friedman SD, et al. Cerebellar vermal volumes and behavioral correlates in children with autism spectrum disorder. Psychiatry 2009;172:61–7.
14. Redcay E, Courchesne E. When is the brain enlarged in autism? A meta-analysis of all brain size reports. Biol Psychiatry 2005;58:1–9.
15. Alexander AL, Lee JE, Lazar M, et al. Diffusion tensor imaging of the corpus callosum in Autism. Neuroimage 2007;34:61–73.
16. Frazier TW, Hardan AY. A meta-analysis of the corpus callosum in autism. Biol Psychiatry 2009; 66:935–41.
17. Spencer MD, Moorhead TW, Lymer GK, et al. Structural correlates of intellectual impairment and autistic features in adolescents. Neuroimage 2006;33:1136–44.
18. Hazlett HC, Poe MD, Gerig G, et al. Cortical gray and white brain tissue volume in adolescents and adults with autism. Biol Psychiatry 2006;59:1–6.
19. Brun CC, Nicolson R, Leporé N, et al. Mapping brain abnormalities in boys with autism. Hum Brain Mapp 2009;30:3887–900.

20. Filipek PA. Quantitative magnetic resonance imaging in autism: the cerebellar vermis. Curr Opin Neurol 1995;8:134–8.
21. Piven J, Saliba K, Bailey J, et al. An MRI study of autism: the cerebellum revisited. Neurology 1997; 49:546–51.
22. Courchesne E, Redcay E, Kennedy DP. The autistic brain: birth through adulthood. Curr Opin Neurol 2004;17:489–96.
23. Monk CS, Peltier SJ, Wiggins JL, et al. Abnormalities of intrinsic functional connectivity in autism spectrum disorders. Neuroimage 2009;47:764–72.
24. Jones TB, Bandettini PA, Kenworthy L, et al. Sources of group differences in functional connectivity: an investigation applied to autism spectrum disorder. Neuroimage 2010;49:401–14.
25. Di Martino A, Ross K, Uddin LQ, et al. Functional brain correlates of social and nonsocial processes in autism spectrum disorders: an activation likelihood estimation meta-analysis. Biol Psychiatry 2009;65:63–74.
26. Thakkar KN, Polli FE, Joseph RM, et al. Response monitoring, repetitive behaviour and anterior cingulate abnormalities in ASD. Brain 2008;131(Pt 9): 2464–78.
27. Ben Bashat D, Kronfeld-Duenias V, Zachor DA, et al. Accelerated maturation of white matter in young children with autism: a high b value DWI study. Neuroimage 2007;37:40–7.
28. Johnstone EC, Crow TJ, Frith CD, et al. Cerebral ventricular size and cognitive impairment in chronic schizophrenia. Lancet 1976;2:924–6.
29. Gur RE, Turetsky BI, Bilker WB, et al. Reduced gray matter volume in schizophrenia. Arch Gen Psychiatry 1999;56:905–11.
30. Park HJ, Levitt J, Shenton ME, et al. An MRI study of spatial probability brain map differences between first-episode schizophrenia and normal controls. Neuroimage 2004;22:1231–46.
31. Davatzikos C, Shen D, Gur RC, et al. Whole-brain morphometric study of schizophrenia revealing a spatially complex set of focal abnormalities. Arch Gen Psychiatry 2005;62:1218–27.
32. Kim JJ, Kim DJ, Kim TG, et al. Volumetric abnormalities in connectivity-based subregions of the thalamus in patients with chronic schizophrenia. Schizophr Res 2007;97:226–35.
33. Glahn DC, Laird AR, Ellison-Wright I, et al. Meta-analysis of gray matter anomalies in schizophrenia: application of anatomic likelihood estimation and network analysis. Biol Psychiatry 2008;64:774–81.
34. Kubicki M, Shenton ME, Salisbury DF, et al. Voxel-based morphometric analysis of gray matter in first episode schizophrenia. Neuroimage 2002;17: 1711–9.
35. Job DE, Whalley HC, McConnell S, et al. Structural gray matter differences between first-episode schizophrenics and normal controls using voxel-based morphometry. Neuroimage 2002;17:880–9.
36. Ellison-Wright I, Bullmore E. Meta-analysis of diffusion tensor imaging studies in schizophrenia. Schizophr Res 2009;108(1–3):3–10.
37. Rametti G, Junqué C, Falcón C, et al. A voxel-based diffusion tensor imaging study of temporal white matter in patients with schizophrenia. Psychiatry Res 2009;171(3):166–76.
38. Kyriakopoulos M, Vyas NS, Barker GJ, et al. A diffusion tensor imaging study of white matter in early-onset schizophrenia. Biol Psychiatry 2008; 63:519–23.
39. Kanaan R, Barker G, Brammer M, et al. White matter microstructure in schizophrenia: effects of disorder, duration and medication. Br J Psychiatry 2009;194:236–42.
40. Nestor PG, Kubicki M, Niznikiewicz M, et al. Neuropsychological disturbance in schizophrenia: a diffusion tensor imaging study. Neuropsychology 2008; 22:246–54.
41. Kawashima T, Nakamura M, Bouix S, et al. Uncinate fasciculus abnormalities in recent onset schizophrenia and affective psychosis: a diffusion tensor imaging study. Schizophr Res 2009;110(1–3):119–26.
42. Oh J, Kubicki M, Rosenberger G, et al. Thalamo-frontal white matter alterations in chronic schizophrenia: a quantitative diffusion tractography study. Hum Brain Mapp 2009;30(11):3812–25.
43. Hubl D, Koenig T, Strik W, et al. Pathways that make voices: white matter changes in auditory hallucinations. Arch Gen Psychiatry 2004;61:658–68.
44. Jones DK, Catani M, Pierpaoli C, et al. Age effects on diffusion tensor magnetic resonance imaging tractography measures of frontal cortex connections in schizophrenia. Hum Brain Mapp 2006;27: 230–8.
45. Dierks T, Linden DE, Jandl M, et al. Activation of Heschl's gyrus during auditory hallucinations. Neuron 1999;22:615–21.
46. Gur RE, Loughead J, Kohler CG, et al. Limbic activation associated with misidentification of fearful faces and flat affect in schizophrenia. Arch Gen Psychiatry 2007;64:1356–66.
47. Camchong J, Macdonald AW, Bell C, et al. Altered functional and anatomical connectivity in schizophrenia. Schizophr Bull 2009. [Epub ahead of print].
48. Huang XQ, Lui S, Deng W, et al. Localization of cerebral functional deficits in treatment-naive, first-episode schizophrenia using resting-state fMRI. Neuroimage 2010;49:2901–6.
49. Allen P, Stephan KE, Mechelli A, et al. Cingulate activity and fronto-temporal connectivity in people with prodromal signs of psychosis. Neuroimage 2010;49:947–55.

50. Rotge JY, Guehl D, Dilharreguy B, et al. Meta-analysis of brain volume changes in obsessive-compulsive disorder. Biol Psychiatry 2009;65:75–83.
51. Radua J, Mataix-Cols D. Voxel-wise meta-analysis of grey matter changes in obsessive-compulsive disorder. Br J Psychiatry 2009;195:393–402.
52. Duran FL, Hoexter MQ, Valente AA, et al. Association between symptom severity and internal capsule volume in obsessive-compulsive disorder. Neurosci Lett 2009;452:68–71.
53. Cannistraro PA, Wright CI, Wedig MM, et al. Amygdala responses to human faces in obsessive-compulsive disorder. Biol Psychiatry 2004;56:916–20.
54. Yoo SY, Jang JH, Shin YW, et al. White matter abnormalities in drug-naïve patients with obsessive-compulsive disorder: a diffusion tensor study before and after citalopram treatment. Acta Psychiatr Scand 2007;116:211–9.
55. Menzies L, Williams GB, Chamberlain SR, et al. White matter abnormalities in patients with obsessive-compulsive disorder and their first-degree relatives. Am J Psychiatry 2008;165(10):1308–15.
56. Nakamae T, Narumoto J, Shibata K, et al. Alteration of fractional anisotropy and apparent diffusion coefficient in obsessive-compulsive disorder: a diffusion tensor imaging study. Prog Neuropsychopharmacol Biol Psychiatry 2008;32(5):1221–6.
57. Szeszko PR, Ardekani BA, Ashtari M, et al. White matter abnormalities in obsessive-compulsive disorder: a diffusion tensor imaging study. Arch Gen Psychiatry 2005;62:782–90.
58. Garibotto V, Scifo P, Gorini A, et al. Disorganization of anatomical connectivity in obsessive compulsive disorder: a multi-parameter diffusion tensor imaging study in a subpopulation of patients. Neurobiol Dis 2010;37(2):468–76.
59. Harrison BJ, Soriano-Mas C, Pujol J, et al. Altered corticostriatal functional connectivity in obsessive-compulsive disorder. Arch Gen Psychiatry 2009;66:1189–200.
60. Roth RM, Saykin AJ, Flashman LA, et al. Event-related functional magnetic resonance imaging of response inhibition in obsessive-compulsive disorder. Biol Psychiatry 2007;62:901–9.
61. Chamberlain SR, Menzies L, Hampshire A, et al. Orbitofrontal dysfunction in patients with obsessive-compulsive disorder and their unaffected relatives. Science 2008;321:421–2.
62. Page LA, Rubia K, Deeley Q, et al. A functional magnetic resonance imaging study of inhibitory control in obsessive-compulsive disorder. Psychiatry Res 2009;174:202–9.
63. An SK, Mataix-Cols D, Lawrence NS, et al. To discard or not to discard: the neural basis of hoarding symptoms in obsessive-compulsive disorder. Mol Psychiatry 2009;14:318–31.
64. Chen CH, Ridler K, Suckling J, et al. Brain imaging correlates of depressive symptom severity and predictors of symptom improvement after antidepressant treatment. Biol Psychiatry 2007;62:407–14.
65. Boes AD, McCormick LM, Coryell WH, et al. Rostral anterior cingulate cortex volume correlates with depressed mood in normal healthy children. Biol Psychiatry 2008;63:391–7.
66. Neumeister A, Wood S, Bonne O, et al. Reduced hippocampal volume in unmedicated, remitted patients with major depression versus control subjects. Biol Psychiatry 2005;57:935–7.
67. Bergouignan L, Chupin M, Czechowska Y, et al. Can voxel based morphometry, manual segmentation and automated segmentation equally detect hippocampal volume differences in acute depression? Neuroimage 2009;45:29–37.
68. Zou K, Deng W, Li T, et al. Changes of brain morphometry in first-episode, drug-naïve, non-late-life adult patients with major depression: an optimized voxel-based morphometry study. Biol Psychiatry 2010;67:186–8.
69. Peterson BS, Warner V, Bansal R, et al. Cortical thinning in persons at increased familial risk for major depression. Proc Natl Acad Sci U S A 2009;106:6273–8.
70. Ma N, Li L, Shu N, et al. White matter abnormalities in first-episode, treatment-naive young adults with major depressive disorder. Am J Psychiatry 2007;164:823–6.
71. Zou K, Huang X, Li T, et al. Alterations of white matter integrity in adults with major depressive disorder: a magnetic resonance imaging study. J Psychiatry Neurosci 2008;33:525–30.
72. Kieseppä T, Eerola M, Mäntylä R, et al. Major depressive disorder and white matter abnormalities: a diffusion tensor imaging study with tract-based spatial statistics. J Affect Disord 2010;120(1–3):240–4.
73. Abe O, Yamasue H, Kasai K, et al. Voxel-based analyses of gray/white matter volume and diffusion tensor data in major depression. Psychiatry Res 2010;181:64–70.
74. Bae JN, Macfall JR, Krishnan KR, et al. Dorsolateral prefrontal cortex and anterior cingulate cortex white matter alterations in late-life depression. Biol Psychiatry 2006;60:1356–63.
75. Yuan Y, Zhang Z, Bai F, et al. White matter integrity of the whole brain is disrupted in first-episode remitted geriatric depression. Neuroreport 2007;18:1845–9.
76. Alexopoulos GS, Murphy CF, Gunning-Dixon FM, et al. Microstructural white matter abnormalities and remission of geriatric depression. Am J Psychiatry 2008;165:238–44.

77. Shimony JS, Sheline YI, D'Angelo G, et al. Diffuse microstructural Abnormalities of normal-appearing white matter in late life depression: a diffusion tensor imaging study. Biol Psychiatry 2009;66(3): 245–52.
78. Frodl T, Bokde AL, Scheuerecker J, et al. Functional connectivity bias of the orbitofrontal cortex in drug-free patients with major depression. Biol Psychiatry 2010;67:161–7.
79. Bluhm R, Williamson P, Lanius R, et al. Resting state default-mode network connectivity in early depression using a seed region-of-interest analysis: decreased connectivity with caudate nucleus. Psychiatry Clin Neurosci 2009;63:754–61.
80. Greicius MD, Flores BH, Menon V, et al. Resting-state functional connectivity in major depression: abnormally increased contributions from subgenual cingulate cortex and thalamus. Biol Psychiatry 2007;62:429–37.
81. Schlösser RG, Wagner G, Koch K, et al. Fronto-cingulate effective connectivity in major depression: a study with fMRI and dynamic causal modeling. Neuroimage 2008;43(3):645–55.
82. Grimm S, Beck J, Schuepbach D, et al. Imbalance between left and right dorsolateral prefrontal cortex in major depression is linked to negative emotional judgment: an fMRI study in severe major depressive disorder. Biol Psychiatry 2008;63:369–76.
83. Penttilä J, Cachia A, Martinot JL, et al. Cortical folding difference between patients with early-onset and patients with intermediate-onset bipolar disorder. Bipolar Disord 2009;11:361–70.
84. Takahashi T, Malhi GS, Wood SJ, et al. Increased pituitary volume in patients with established bipolar affective disorder. Prog Neuropsychopharmacol Biol Psychiatry 2009;33:1245–9.
85. Savitz J, Nugent AC, Bogers W, et al. Amygdala volume in depressed patients with bipolar disorder assessed using high resolution 3T MRI: the impact of medication. Neuroimage 2010;49(4):2966–76.
86. Bearden CE, Thompson PM, Dalwani M, et al. Greater cortical gray matter density in lithium-treated patients with bipolar disorder. Biol Psychiatry 2007;62:7–16.
87. Kempton MJ, Geddes JR, Ettinger U, et al. Meta-analysis, database, and meta-regression of 98 structural imaging studies in bipolar disorder. Arch Gen Psychiatry 2008;65:1017–32.
88. Arnone D, Cavanagh J, Gerber D, et al. Magnetic resonance imaging studies in bipolar disorder and schizophrenia: meta-analysis. Br J Psychiatry 2009;195:194–201.
89. Lloyd AJ, Moore PB, Cousins DA, et al. White matter lesions in euthymic patients with bipolar disorder. Acta Psychiatr Scand 2009;120:481–91.
90. Vita A, De Peri L, Sacchetti E. Gray matter, white matter, brain, and intracranial volumes in first-episode bipolar disorder: a meta-analysis of magnetic resonance imaging studies. Bipolar Disord 2009;11:807–14.
91. Macritchie KA, Lloyd AJ, Bastin ME, et al. White matter microstructural abnormalities in euthymic bipolar disorder. Br J Psychiatry 2010;196:52–8.
92. Adler CM, Holland SK, Schmithorst V, et al. Abnormal frontal white matter tracts in bipolar disorder: a diffusion tensor imaging study. Bipolar Disord 2004;6:197–203.
93. Haznedar MM, Roversi F, Pallanti S, et al. Fronto-thalamo-striatal gray and white matter volumes and anisotropy of their connections in bipolar spectrum illnesses. Biol Psychiatry 2005;57:733–42.
94. Beyer JL, Taylor WD, MacFall JR, et al. Cortical white matter microstructural abnormalities in bipolar disorder. Neuropsychopharmacology 2005;30:2225–9.
95. Yurgelun-Todd DA, Silveri MM, Gruber SA, et al. White matter abnormalities observed in bipolar disorder: a diffusion tensor imaging study. Bipolar Disord 2007;9:504–12.
96. Houenou J, Wessa M, Douaud G, et al. Increased white matter connectivity in euthymic bipolar patients: diffusion tensor tractography between the subgenual cingulate and the amygdalo-hippocampal complex. Mol Psychiatry 2007; 12:1001–10.
97. Versace A, Almeida JR, Hassel S, et al. Elevated left and reduced right orbitomedial prefrontal fractional anisotropy in adults with bipolar disorder revealed by tract-based spatial statistics. Arch Gen Psychiatry 2008;65:1041–52.
98. Wessa M, Houenou J, Leboyer M, et al. Microstructural white matter changes in euthymic bipolar patients: a whole-brain diffusion tensor imaging study. Bipolar Disord 2009;11:504–14.
99. Wang F, Kalmar JH, He Y, et al. Functional and structural connectivity between the perigenual anterior cingulate and amygdala in bipolar disorder. Biol Psychiatry 2009;66:516–21.
100. Almeida JR, Mechelli A, Hassel S, et al. Abnormally increased effective connectivity between parahippocampal gyrus and ventromedial prefrontal regions during emotion labeling in bipolar disorder. Psychiatry Res 2009;174:195–201.
101. Rich BA, Vinton DT, Roberson-Nay R, et al. Limbic hyperactivation during processing of neutral facial expressions in children with bipolar disorder. Proc Natl Acad Sci U S A 2006;103:8900–5.
102. Robinson JL, Bearden CE, Monkul ES, et al. Fronto-temporal dysregulation in remitted bipolar patients: an fMRI delayed-non-match-to-sample (DNMS) study. Bipolar Disord 2009;11:351–60.
103. Gruber O, Tost H, Henseler I, et al. Pathological amygdala activation during working memory performance: evidence for a pathophysiological

trait marker in bipolar affective disorder. Hum Brain Mapp 2010;31:115–25.
104. Glahn DC, Robinson JL, Tordesillas-Gutierrez D, et al. Fronto-temporal dysregulation in asymptomatic bipolar I patients: a paired associate functional MRI study. Hum Brain Mapp 2010. [Epub ahead of print].
105. Dalton KM, Nacewicz BM, Alexander AL, et al. Gaze-fixation, brain activation, and amygdala volume in unaffected siblings of individuals with autism. Biol Psychiatry 2007;61:512–20.
106. Greimel E, Schulte-Rüther M, Kircher T, et al. Neural mechanisms of empathy in adolescents with autism spectrum disorder and their fathers. Neuroimage 2010;49:1055–65.
107. Ohnishi T, Hashimoto R, Mori T, et al. The association between the Val158Met polymorphism of the catechol-O-methyl transferase gene and morphological abnormalities of the brain in chronic schizophrenia. Brain 2006;129:399–410.
108. Honea R, Verchinski BA, Pezawas L, et al. Impact of interacting functional variants in COMT on regional gray matter volume in human brain. Neuroimage 2009;45:44–51.
109. Narr KL, Szeszko PR, Lencz T, et al. DTNBP1 is associated with imaging phenotypes in schizophrenia. Hum Brain Mapp 2009;30:3783–94.
110. Egan MF, Goldberg TE, Kolachana BS, et al. Effect of COMT Val108/158 Met genotype on frontal lobe function and risk for schizophrenia. Proc Natl Acad Sci U S A 2001;98:6917–22.
111. Straub RE, Lipska BK, Egan MF, et al. Allelic variation in GAD1 (GAD67) is associated with schizophrenia and influences cortical function and gene expression. Mol Psychiatry 2007;12:854–69.
112. Mechelli A, Prata DP, Fu CH, et al. The effects of neuregulin1 on brain function in controls and patients with schizophrenia and bipolar disorder. Neuroimage 2008;42:817–26.
113. Soriano-Mas C, Pujol J, Alonso P, et al. Identifying patients with obsessive-compulsive disorder using whole-brain anatomy. Neuroimage 2007;35: 1028–37.
114. Caprihan A, Pearlson GD, Calhoun VD. Application of principal component analysis to distinguish patients with schizophrenia from healthy controls based on fractional anisotropy measurements. Neuroimage 2008;42(2):675–82.
115. Sun D, van Erp TG, Thompson PM, et al. Elucidating a magnetic resonance imaging-based neuroanatomic biomarker for psychosis: classification analysis using probabilistic brain atlas and machine learning algorithms. Biol Psychiatry 2009;66:1055–60.
116. Nenadic I, Sauer H, Gaser C. Distinct pattern of brain structural deficits in subsyndromes of schizophrenia delineated by psychopathology. Neuroimage 2010;49:1153–60.
117. Fan Y, Gur RE, Gur RC, et al. Unaffected family members and schizophrenia patients share brain structure patterns: a high-dimensional pattern classification study. Biol Psychiatry 2008;63:118–24.
118. Jenike MA, Baer L, Ballantine T, et al. Cingulotomy for refractory obsessive-compulsive disorder. A long-term follow-up of 33 patients. Arch Gen Psychiatry 1991;48:548–55.
119. Rück C, Karlsson A, Steele JD, et al. Capsulotomy for obsessive-compulsive disorder: long-term follow-up of 25 patients. Arch Gen Psychiatry 2008;65:914–21.
120. Mayberg HS. Targeted electrode-based modulation of neural circuits for depression. J Clin Invest 2009;119:717–25.
121. Gutman DA, Holtzheimer PE, Behrens TE, et al. A tractography analysis of two deep brain stimulation white matter targets for depression. Biol Psychiatry 2009; 65(4):276–82.

PET in Brain Tumors

Roland Hustinx, MD, PhD*, Pacôme Fosse, MD

KEYWORDS

- Brain tumors • Positron emission tomography
- 18F-fluorodeoxyglucose • Methyl-L-methionine • FET

In 2009, the estimated number of new cases of primary tumors of the brain and other nervous system was 22,070 in the United States.[1] The estimated number of deaths was 12,920. The incidence of primary brain tumors is increasing in association with the ageing of the general population. Metastases to the central nervous system are far more frequent, but PET imaging of such involvement is beyond the scope of this article. Tumors of the central nervous system are classified according to the World Health Organization (WHO) system, which was revised in 2007.[2] A summarized version of this classification is shown in **Box 1**. In addition to the pathologic type, the WHO classification also provides a histologic grade, w hich tends to assess the malignancy scale of the lesion and characterize its biologic behavior. Although widely used and recognized as a major factor in the clinical management, the grading scheme is not mandatory for applying the WHO classification. Grade 1 lesions display low proliferative potential, and complete surgical resection alone may cure the patients. Grade 2 lesions also have a low proliferative pattern but are often bound to recur because of their 2infiltrative nature. Some grade 2 lesions such as astrocytomas, oligoastrocytomas, and oligodendrogliomas also may transform into aggressive forms over time. Grade 3 tumors display malignant features such as nuclear atypia and enhanced mitotic activity. Grade 4 lesions are the most aggressive with rapid clinical progression. These tumors are highly infiltrative and often largely necrotic. The most common example of grade 4 tumor is the glioblastoma.[2] Treatment options and prognosis greatly vary depending on the tumor type and grade, location in the brain, which also contributes determining the resectability of the lesion, and age of the patient. The most frequent primary neoplasms of the central nervous system (CNS) are the tumors of neuroepithelial tissue, in particular astrocytic tumors, followed by the meningiomas.

Magnetic resonance imaging (MRI) with gadolinium contrast enhancement is considered the imaging gold standard in the diagnosis and follow-up of primary CNS tumors. It provides anatomic details of exquisitely high precision, and functional information such as vascular permeability, cell density, and tumor perfusion. Overall, MRI has an excellent sensitivity in these indications, but it also has several limitations. It cannot always distinguish gliomas from non-neoplastic lesions such as inflammatory or vascular processes. Discriminating peritumoral vasogenic edema and tumoral infiltration of this edema is often difficult. MRI is also imperfect for grading gliomas, as the absence of contrast enhancement does not always correspond to a low-grade tumor. Furthermore, distinguishing tumor recurrence from post-therapeutic changes remains challenging. In meningiomas, bone involvement is better depicted using computed tomography (CT) than MRI. The field is rapidly evolving, however, as advanced MRI modalities in particular using diffusion and perfusion-weighted sequences increasingly are used and perfected, substantially improving the specificity of the test.[3]

PET TRACERS FOR BRAIN TUMOR IMAGING

18F-fluorodeoxyglucose (FDG) remains the most widely used PET tracer in oncology, including neuro-oncology. Tumor cells suffer deep biochemical changes, specific to the malignant transformation

Division of Nuclear Medicine, University Hospital of Liège, University of Liège, B35, 4000 Liège I, Belgium
* Corresponding author.
E-mail address: rhustinx@chu.ulg.ac.be

PET Clin 5 (2010) 185–197
doi:10.1016/j.cpet.2010.02.004
1556-8598/10/$ – see front matter

Box 1
Tumor types

Tumors of neuroepithelial tissue

- Astrocytic tumors
  - Pilocytic astrocytoma
  - Subependymal giant cell astrocytoma
  - Pleomorphic xanthoastrocytoma
  - Diffuse astrocytoma
  - Anaplastic astrocytoma
  - Glioblastoma
  - Gliomatosis cerebri
- Oligodendroglial tumors
  - Oligodendroglioma
  - Anaplastic oligodendroglioma
- Olioastrocytic tumors
  - Oligoastrocytoma
  - Anaplastic oligoastrocytoma
- Ependymal tumors
  - Subependymoma
  - Myxopapillary ependymoma
  - Ependymoma
  - Anaplastic ependymoma
- Choroid plexus tumors
  - Choroid plexus papilloma
  - Atypical choroid plexus papilloma
  - Choroid plexus carcinoma
- Other neuroepithelial tumors
  - Astroblastoma
  - Chordoid glioma of the third ventricle
  - Angiocentric glioma
- Neuronal and mixed neuronal–glial tumors
- Tumors of the pineal region
- Embryonal tumors
  - Medulloblastoma
  - CNS primitive neuroectodermal tumor
  - Atypical teratoid/rhabdoid tumor

Tumors of cranial and paraspinal nerves

- Schwannoma (neurilemoma, neurinoma)
- Neurofibroma
- Perineurioma
- Malignant peripheral

Tumors of the meninges

- Tumors of meningothelial cells
  - Meningioma
- Mesenchymal tumors
- Primary melanocytic lesions
- Other neoplasms related to the meninges

Lymphomas and hematopoietic neoplasms

Germ cell tumors

Tumors of the sellar region

Metastatic tumors

and not solely related to the accelerated growth rate. Increased glycolytic rates result from various processes including high levels of enzymes that control glycolysis such as hexokinase, phosphofructokinase, and pyruvate dehydrogenase and increased membrane glucose transport capability. PET therefore can take advantage from this increased capacity for glucose transport observed in malignant glial cells to image brain tumors with FDG.[4–6] As discussed later, the relationship between FDG uptake, tumor type and tumor type is complex. It generally is considered, however, that FDG uptake reflects the burden of tumor cell viability and density, and is directly related with the tumor grade, as suggested by early works by Di Chiro and colleagues[7] and Herholz and colleagues.[8] FDG PET imaging goes further than simply exploring metabolic pathways. It provides unique information regarding key molecular changes arising in tumor cells. For instance, a relationship recently was shown between FDG uptake and 1p and 19q loss of heterozygosity (1p/19q LOH) in WHO grade 2 gliomas.[9] Such observations may be highly clinically relevant, as 1p/19q LOH is associated with a favorable prognosis and response to chemotherapy and radiation therapy in oligodendroglial tumors. Another example is the relationship between the mammalian target of rapamycin (mTOR) activity and FDG uptake. mTOR is a key signaling molecule involved in the growth of glioblastoma among others, and it has become a potential biologic target for treating these tumors.[10] Preclinical data showed inhibition of hexokinase activity and reduced FDG uptake in human glioma cell lines that were sensitive to rapamycin.[11] These changes were observed as early as 24 hours after starting the treatment.

The high physiologic activity of the normal cortex must be taken into account when using FDG PET for imaging brain tumors. Unlike other locations in the body, the contrast between the tumor and surrounding normal tissue may be limited, including for FDG-avid lesions. Quantifying FDG uptake is of limited value, and the interpretation of the scan usually relies upon visual analysis in correlation with MRI findings and assessment of the metabolic ratios (ie, the tumor-to-normal contralateral white matter [T/WM] or the tumor-to-cortex [T/C] activity ratios).[12,13] Standardized uptake values (SUV) are poorly correlated with regional metabolic rates of glucose use (MRGlu), and are less effective in characterizing primary brain tumors than tumor-to-white matter or T/C activity ratios.[14]

In contrast with FDG, amino acid analogs are not significantly taken up by the normal cortex. The first tracer of this class and the best known is ^{11}C-methyl-L-methionine (MET).[15] It is easily synthesized, but its main drawback relates to the short half-life of the carbon-11.[16] Fluorinated analogs were developed, and several are available, including O-(2-^{18}F-fluoroethyl)-L-tyrosine (FET), 2-^{18}F-fluoro-L-tyrosine (F-TYR), L-3-^{18}F-alpha-methyl tyrosine (FMT), and 3,4-dihydroxy-6-^{18}F-fluoro-l-phenylalanine (F-DOPA).[17–20] MET is incorporated into newly formed protein, but its uptake process is complex and related to both the protein synthesis rate and amino acid transport. It also is incorporated into phospholipids,[21] however, and a passive diffusion in tumors with breakdown of the blood–brain barrier was reported to contribute to tracer accumulation.[22] The tumor uptake of the fluorinated tyrosine derivatives is more directly related to the transport of amino acids, especially the LAT-1 subsystem for F-TYR[23] and the LAT-2 subsystem for FET.[24] Despite the differences existing between the precise molecular mechanisms of uptake of the various radiolabeled amino acid analogs, and even though there are no large clinical series comparing these tracers side by side, it appears that for most of the common indications, very similar patterns of uptake are expected.[25]

FDG and amino acid analogs are the most widely used tracers for brain tumor imaging with PET, but other compounds also have been investigated with potential specific clinical application. 3′-fluoro-3′-deoxythymidine (FLT) is a fluorinated nucleoside that is intracellularly phosphorylated by the thymidine kinase TK1. As TK1 activity is cell cycle dependant and frequently overexpressed in proliferating tumor cells, the uptake of FLT is directly proportional to DNA synthesis and cell proliferation.[26] Similar to amino acid analogs, the FLT uptake by the normal brain is very low, which makes it an attractive option for neuroimaging. Choline is a quaternary ammonium base, of which several analogs are available, labeled with either F18 or C11.[27–29] The cell malignant transformation is associated with increased activity of the choline kinase, related to tumor proliferation and increased need for cytoplasmic membrane constituents.[30] Finally, the somatostatin analog DOTA (0)-D-Phe (1)-Tyr (3)-octreotide (DOTATOC) can be labeled with 68Ga, a positron-emitting radionuclide with a physical half-life of 68 minutes. As the radiosynthesis is fairly straightforward and given that 68Ga is available through an on-site generator, DOTATOC has generated great interest among research groups.[31] Of particular interest is the fact that meningiomas have been shown to express somatostatin receptors both in vitro and in vivo, which led to successful PET imaging with DOTATOC, with low background activity.[32]

CLINICAL APPLICATIONS

Diagnosis and Characterization of Brain Tumors

In gliomas, the relationship between the intensity of FDG uptake and tumor grade has been largely documented.[7,12,33,34] As a general rule, a level of FDG uptake approaching or superior to the contralateral gray matter corresponds to grade 3 and 4 tumors, whereas a level of uptake close to that of the white matter indicates a low-grade lesion. There are notable exceptions, however, as pilocytic astrocytomas and low-grade oligodendrogliomas may display highly increased FDG uptake.[33] Kosaka and colleagues[35] studied 34 patients selected according to radiologic criteria. All presented with nodular enhancement greater than 1 cm in diameter or ring enhancement greater than 1 cm thick in the marginal solid portion. All primary malignant tumors showed greatly increased uptake,with the highest being observed in lymphomas (T/Cmax 3,29 on average, as compared with 1,71 for high grade gliomas). Metastases from various primaries showed a somewhat lower uptake, but the limited sensitivity of PET for detecting such lesions is known.[36,37] Combined with MRI, FDG PET may be considered, when highly hyperactive, as a fairly good indicator of the presence of an aggressive lesion. Because of the high cortical uptake, lesions with mild-to-moderate uptake may be missed altogether, especially when the MRI study is not available to guide the PET reading. As a result, the overall sensitivity of FDG-PET is quite low, in particular for low-grade gliomas.

The absence of uptake in the normal cortex constitutes a significant advantage of radiolabeled amino acid analogs over FDG, as it allows for a better delineation of the tumor boundaries, including in lo- grade gliomas. However, even though the sensitivity for detecting such lesions is higher than with FDG, it remains far from perfect. In a series of 50 patients with gliomas, MET uptake was increased in 31 of 32 high-grade lesions and 11 of 18 low-grade lesions.[38] Other studies report slightly higher sensitivities, ranging from 76% to 87%, and a specificity ranging from 75% to 89% for diagnosing untreated brain tumors.[39–42] A recent study dealing with children and young adults found an 83% sensitivity and a 92% specificity using a threshold of 1,48 for the T/C activity ratios.[43] Similar figures are reported regarding the sensitivity of FET, which is the most extensively investigated fluorinated amino acid analog.[44,45] Floeth and colleagues[46] cautioned against the possibly limited specificity of FET-PET in characterizing lesions that show ring enhancement on MRI, as it was positive in three of nine patients with benign conditions (abscess or demyelinating lesion). High sensitivities also were reported with FDOPA, although the published series involve mixed patients populations, with a minority of untreated cases.[47,48] Nonetheless, as far as sensitivity is concerned, amino acid analogs are clearly superior to FDG for diagnosing low- and high-grade gliomas.

The relationship between intensity of amino acid analog uptake and tumor grade remains subject to speculations. Results with MET are conflicting, as some investigators found a good correlation between the two parameters,[49–51] while others reached the opposite conclusion.[33,52,53] Similarly, most studies failed to reliably classify gliomas according to their WHO pathologic grade, based upon the level of FET uptake.[45,54] It seems, however, that the uptake kinetics differs among low- and high-grade gliomas, as a slight increase over time is observed in the former, compared with an early peak followed by a decrease in the later.[55]

Along with a better characterization of the tumor grade, FDG PET also is associated with a stronger prognostic value than amino acids, as a high FDG uptake strongly indicates shorter survival.[45,56,57] Of particular clinical interest are those patients with FDG-avid low-grade gliomas, as they appear to behave differently from the cold lesions with similar histology. Unfavorable clinical evolution of such lesions has been reported in adults and in children.[58,59] Such observations do not translate into clinical practice yet, but a metabolic risk stratification may lead to improved, risk-based, treatment algorithms for selected subgroups of patients. Similarly, and although FDG performs better across all types and grades of astrocytic tumors, combining MRI features with FET results in selected subgroups of homogeneous patients may yield clinically relevant prognostic information. Among the body of work performed by the Jülich group, Floeth and colleagues[60] studied 33 patients with grade 2 gliomas, mainly astrocytomas. Patients with circumscribed lesions on MRI and no FET uptake had the best prognosis, whereas those with diffuse MRI lesions with FET uptake showed all rapid progression or malignant transformation. **Figs. 1** and **2** show examples of low-grade gliomas.

In spite of these positive results, the prognostic value of metabolic imaging is not such as histologic assessment of the lesions could be withheld. Much more than imaging results, pathologic analysis remains a key parameter guiding the therapeutic strategy. In this setting, PET may be helpful in identifying target biopsy sites, thus enhancing the diagnostic yield of this invasive procedure. This was proposed as early as 1991 by Hanson and colleagues,[61] with FDG-PET, and further developed by other researchers, in particular the group at the Free University of Brussels.[62] Combining FDG and MET, they found that in patients with increased uptake of both tracers, the focus of highest MET uptake corresponds to the focus of highest FDG uptake, even though the extent of uptake of both tracers is variable.[63] Out of 70 biopsy trajectories, all 61 MET-positive trajectories yielded a diagnosis of tumor, whereas the nondiagnostic procedures were found in regions with no MET uptake. Compared with MRI alone, PET improves the diagnostic yield and reduces the number of sampling procedures, including in complex situations such as brainstem lesions in children.[64] These procedures are methodologically and logistically demanding, and such impressive results only can be achieved in centers with experienced and well-coordinated interdisciplinary teams.

Most of the results discussed previously dealt with tumors of neuroepithelial tissue, in particular astrocytic or oligodendroglial tumors. Meningiomas are the second most frequent tumors encountered in the brain, and PET recently has drawn interest for characterizing these lesions. Most, but not all meningiomas are low-grade tumors, and the recurrence rate after treatment is related directly to the tumor grade, up to 73% in patients with WHO grade 3 lesions.[65] Meningiomas usually do not accumulate FDG, but a relationship between tumor aggressivity and presence of FDG uptake was reported by several groups.[66,67] Even considering grade 3 meningiomas only, the sensitivity of FDG-PET remains very low, 43% in a recent report,[68] so that the value of the test lies in the tumor characterization and prediction of its recurrence rather than in its

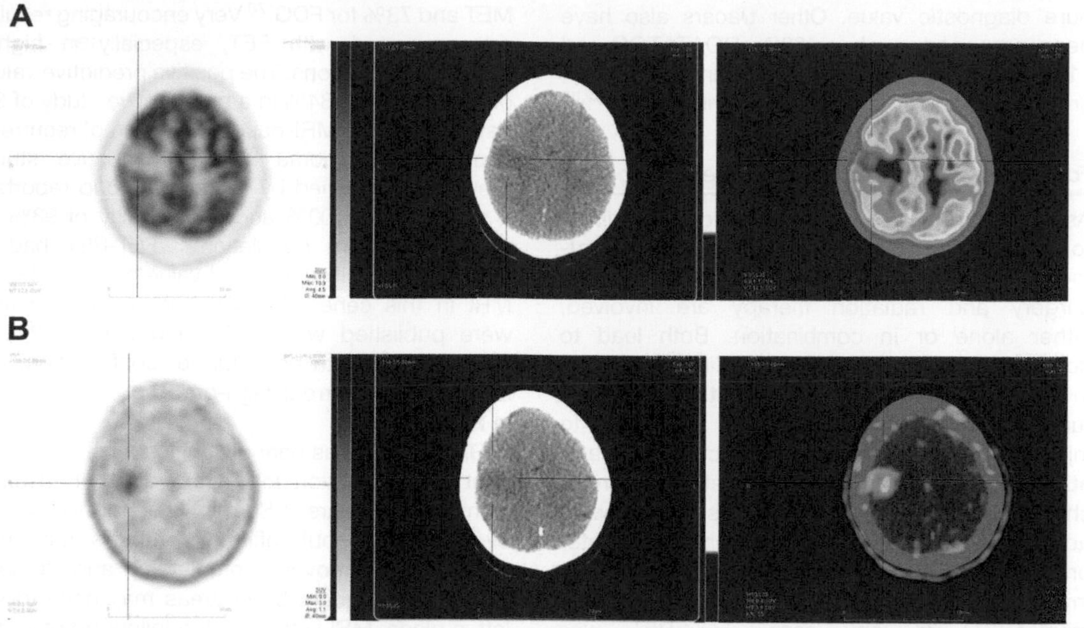

Fig. 1. This 37-year-old had a neurologic evaluation following seizures. Magnetic resonance imaging (MRI) showed an infiltrative lesion of the right Rolandic area. FDG PET/CT showed an area of decreased uptake, with a T/C activity ratio of 0.5 (*A*). There was a significant uptake of F-TYR in the corresponding area, with a T/C activity ratio of 1.7 (*B*). A stereotaxic biopsy revealed a World Health Organization (WHO) grade 2 oligodendroglioma.

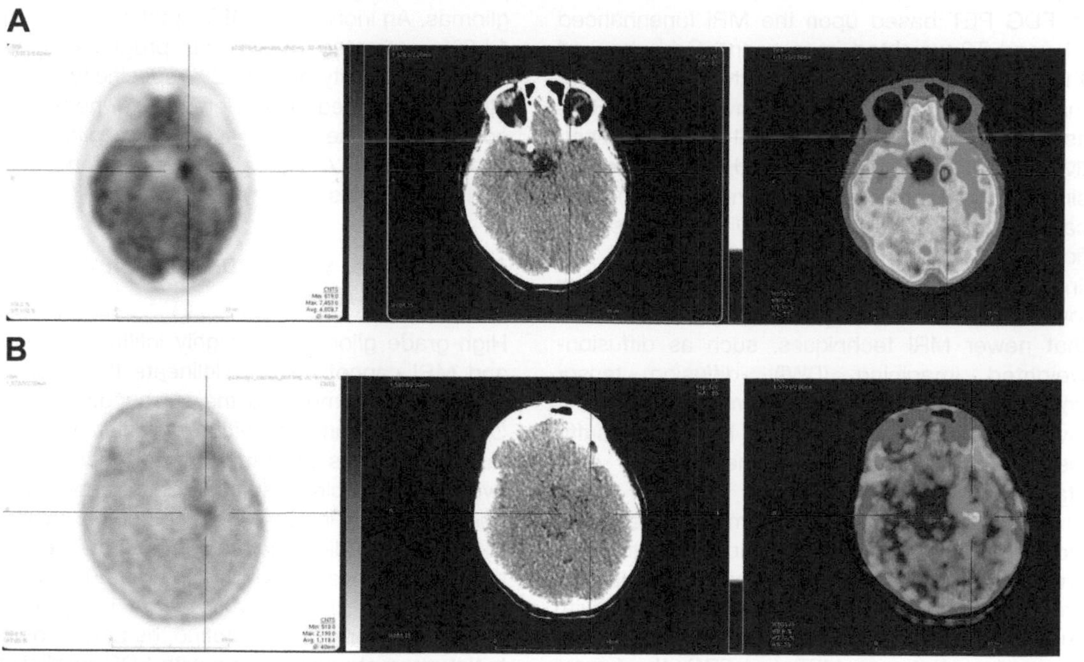

Fig. 2. This 36-year-old woman was diagnosed with a left temporal lobe fibrillary astrocytoma, WHO grade 2. The pathologic examination of the biopsy samples also showed a proliferative index of 10%, which is unusually high for such tumor. The FDG PET study showed a focus of increased activity in the deep temporal lobe (*A*), which corresponds to an increased uptake of F-TYR (*B*). Ten months later, surgery was performed because of clinical and radiological progression. Pathology revealed a glioblastoma.

pure diagnostic value. Other tracers also have been proposed, such as 68Ga-DOATATOC and 11C-choline, which show high tumor to background contrast even in grade 1 meningiomas.[32,69]

Follow-up of Treated or Untreated Tumors

As mentioned earlier, various factors contribute to the decision to treat and the choice of treatment scheme in gliomas. Very often, however, surgery and radiation therapy are involved, either alone or in combination. Both lead to nonspecific changes in MRI findings, resulting in a low specificity for detecting recurrent tumors. Irradiation of the brain may lead to injuries that are often loosely described as radiation necrosis. The term radiation necrosis should be reserved to those lesions showing actual necrosis, usually corresponding to late-onset irreversible injuries (months to years after irradiation) as opposed to earlier, reversible injuries.[70,71] In any case, FDG-PET was proposed very early on as a tool for differentiating recurrence from radiation injuries. Since the initial report by Patronas and colleagues[72] in 1982, a fairly large literature has been made available. Results are somewhat conflicting, however, and methodological issues limit the level of evidence provided by many of these papers. Prior selection of the patients submitted to FDG PET based upon the MRI (unenhanced T1- and T2-weighted images and Gd-enhanced T1-weighted images) is mandatory, considering that the major limitation of conventional MRI is its limited specificity, whereas it is highly sensitive. In these patients, increased FDG uptake (ie, similar or superior to the normal cortex) indicates tumor recurrence with a high specificity.[73,74] Sensitivity is an issue, however, not limited to the low-grade gliomas, as values as low as 40% were reported.[75] It should be noted that newer MRI techniques, such as diffusion-weighted imagining (DWI), diffusion tensor imaging (DTI), and perfusion imaging are being investigated. None, however, has been sufficiently validated as to become the new gold standard.[76]

Because of these limitations, most of the recent works focused on alternative tracers, in particular amino acid analogs. MET showed 75% sensitivity and 75% specificity in a series of 26 patients with suspected recurrent gliomas.[77] In a direct comparison between MET and FDG, the former was found to be superior, as it showed pathologically increased uptake in 28 of 30 scans, as compared with 17 of 30 scans with FDG. Interestingly, the interobserver agreement was 100% for MET and 73% for FDG.[78] Very encouraging results were reported with FET, especially in highly selected populations. The positive predictive value of FET-PET was 84% in a prospective study of 31 patients with an MRI-based suspicion of recurrent supratentorial glioma.[79] A retrospective study previously published by the same group reported a sensitivity of 100% and a specificity of 93% in a similar patient population.[80] FET-PET had a statistically significant added value compared with MRI in this series. Equally encouraging results were published with FLT[81] and FDOPA,[48] but these limited data need further confirmation. An example of recurrent high-grade glioma is given in **Fig. 3**.

Grade 2 gliomas bear a significant risk of malignant transformation into grade 3 or 4, usually within 5 to 10 years.[82] Surgery is performed whenever possible, but infiltrative tumors may not always be removed completely, and tumors located in eloquent brain areas may have to be left in place. MRI is used in the follow-up of these patients, but in many cases it cannot clearly identify malignant progression. PET thus may be helpful in patients with alarming clinical signs and inconclusive MRI findings. FDG initially was proposed in this setting,[83] but amino acid analogs again seem to be the preferred tracers. Ullrich and colleagues[84] repeatedly performed MET PET in 24 patients with grade 2 (n = 18) or grade 3 (n = 6) gliomas. An increase in MET uptake of more than 14.6% indicated malignant progression with a 90% sensitivity and a 92% specificity. Further studies are needed to determine whether PET could be of use in the systematic follow-up of such patients. A typical example of malignant transformation is shown in **Fig. 4**.

PET for Target Volume Delineation in Radiation Therapy

High-grade gliomas are highly infiltrating lesions and MRI cannot reliably delineate the boundary between the tumor and the surrounding edema. On the other hand, definition of radiation therapy target volume is of primary importance. Indeed, even though a clear radiation dose response has been observed in experimental studies, randomized clinical studies failed to demonstrate a translation into improved survival.[85] In brain tumors as in other tumors, there is a trend to integrate the metabolic information to define the target volume. Initial attempts were made with FDG in glioblastoma, showing that the metabolic volume was significantly different from the MRI volume and that the former was more predictive for survival and time to progression after radiation therapy

A

B

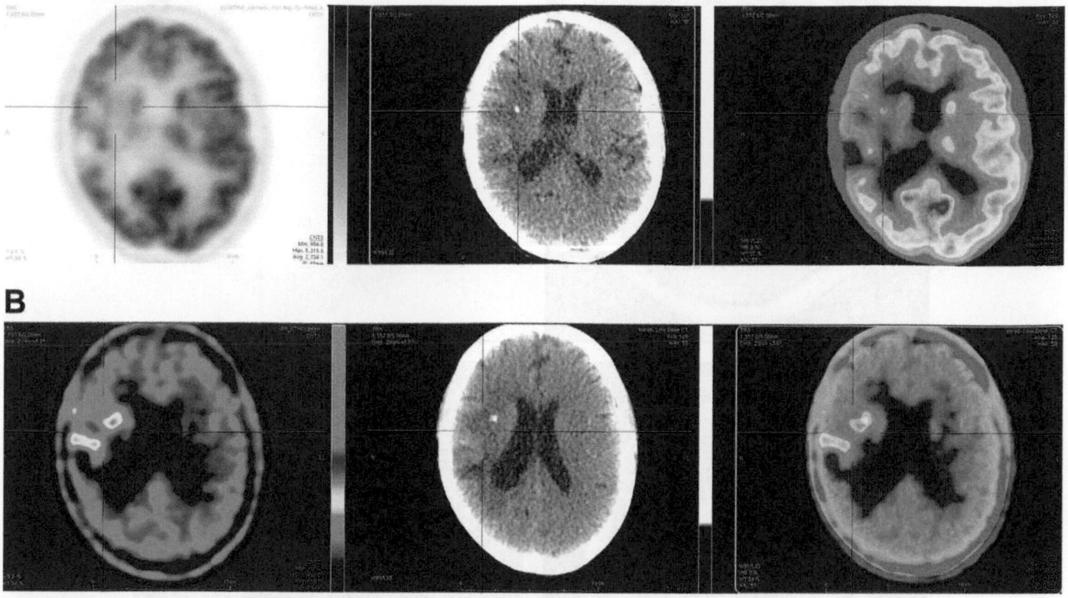

Fig. 3. A 60-year-old man was treated by surgery and radiation therapy for a glioblastoma. During the follow-up, a recurrence was suspected based upon MRI changes. PET/CT with FDG showed an heterogeneous uptake in the controversial area of the brain, difficult to distinguish from cortex (*A*). The F-TYR scan showed two foci of highly increased uptake, consistent with relapse, which was confirmed by the clinical evolution.

than the latter.[86,87] Grosu and colleagues[88] investigated MET in this indication and found high discrepancies in tumor volumes according to the reference method. In 5 of 39 patients (13%), MET uptake corresponded exactly with Gd enhancement, whereas in 29 of 39 patients (74%), the region of MET uptake was larger than that of the Gd enhancement. In 27 (69%) of the 39 patients, the Gd enhancement area extended beyond the MET enhancement. All patients were imaged after surgery, which is not the ideal situation for MRI. Similar results were found by Mahasittiwat and colleagues[89] in a smaller series. Major changes in target volumes also were observed with FET-PET in patients with glioblastoma.[85,90] Although a good concordance was observed between the biologic volumes manually delineated by three independent observers,[90] methodological questions persist in regard to the optimal way for segmenting the PET images. Also, at this point, the real clinical impact of integrating the biologic information into the irradiation treatment planning remains totally unknown and will remain so until interventional studies are conducted.

Meningiomas also are treated frequently by a combination of surgery and radiation therapy, as postoperative irradiation improves the local control and diminishes the risk of regrowth. Radiation therapy in this setting has become highly conformational, and meningiomas, especially those located at the base of the skull, present with specific challenges when it comes to defining the target volume. Both CT and MRI are used because of the usefulness of combining the superior soft tissue imaging afforded by MRI with the geometric accuracy of CT. Identifying bone involvement is often difficult, whatever the cross-sectional imaging technique used. Both amino acid analogs and DOTATOC have been proposed in this setting, with similar end results. DOTATOC changed the target volume in 65% (17 of 26) and 73% (19 of 26) of the published cases.[91,92] In a pilot study of 13 patients, the extent of the anomalies according to F-TYR PET/CT and MRI differed in approximately half the cases (6 of 13 tumors).[93] In most cases, the discrepancy resulted from a larger extent measured on PET than on MRI. Grosu and colleagues used MET in 10 meningiomas at the base of the skull and found metabolic changes in a similar proportion (60%), but in these patients, the addition of 11C-MET tended to reduce the target volume (40% of the cases) rather than increase it (20% of the cases).[94] In any case, these preliminary results emphasize the high clinical impact that might stem from integrating the metabolic information, as all studies without

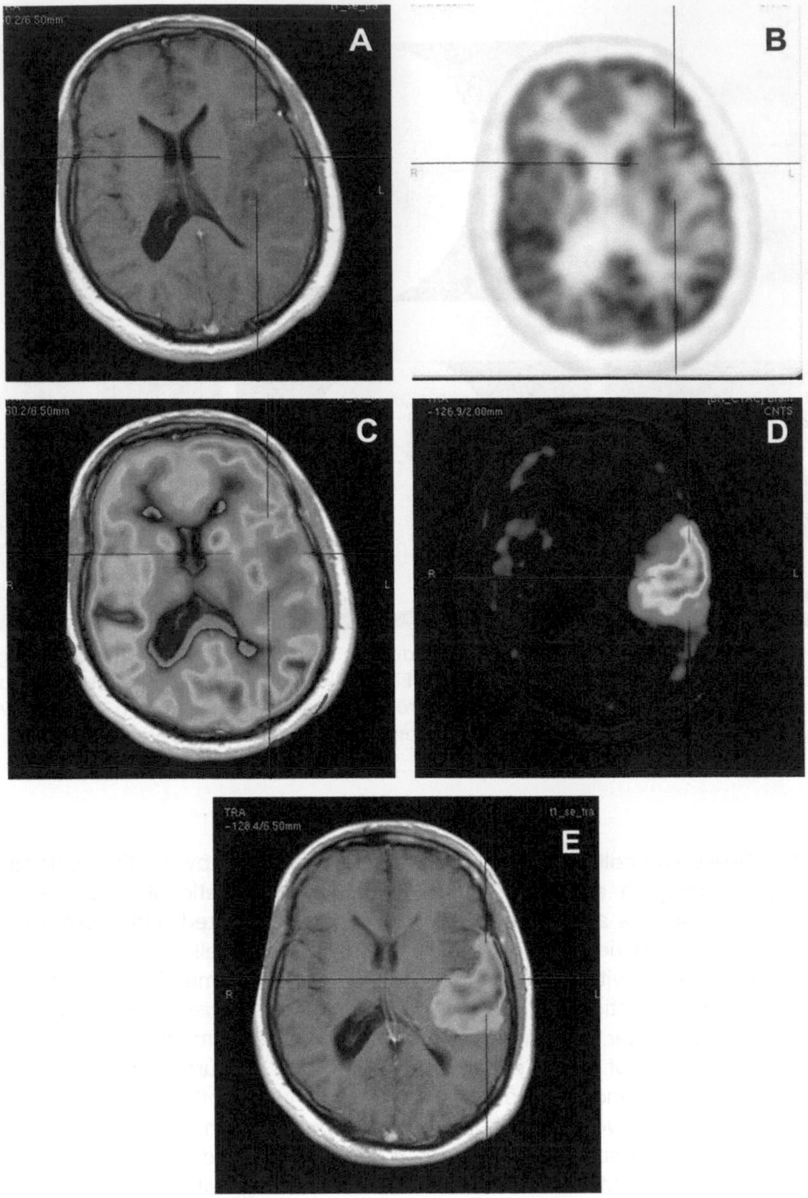

Fig. 4. This 31-year-old man had a known low-grade glioma that had been stable for 6 years. The MRI remained unchanged, showing a diffuse infiltrative lesion in the left parietotemporal area, without Gd enhancement on the T1w-images (*A*). FDG PET showed a heterogeneous uptake in the area, with a level of activity similar to the normal cortex (*B*: FDG, *C*: fused FDG/MRI). The F-TYR PET scan showed highly increased uptake in the entire lesion, with a T/C activity ratio of 3.1 (*D*: F-TYR, *E*: fused F-TYR/MRI). Based upon these findings, a biopsy was performed, revealing a glioblastoma.

exception report significant changes in volume and geometric distribution of the tumor in most patients. An example of meningioma of the base of the skull is shown in **Fig. 5**.

PET for Evaluating the Response to Treatment

Data remain scarce regarding the usefulness of PET in the evaluation of treatment response. Currently, temozolomide, an orally given alkylating agent, is often prescribed as an adjuvant treatment to patients with glioblastoma and anaplastic astrocytoma, leading to slightly improved survival, at least in the glioblastoma patients.[95] In a pilot study, Brock and colleagues[96] demonstrated that a 25% reduction in the region of highest uptake (measured as the MRGlu, but not the SUV) with FDG-PET could differentiate responders from

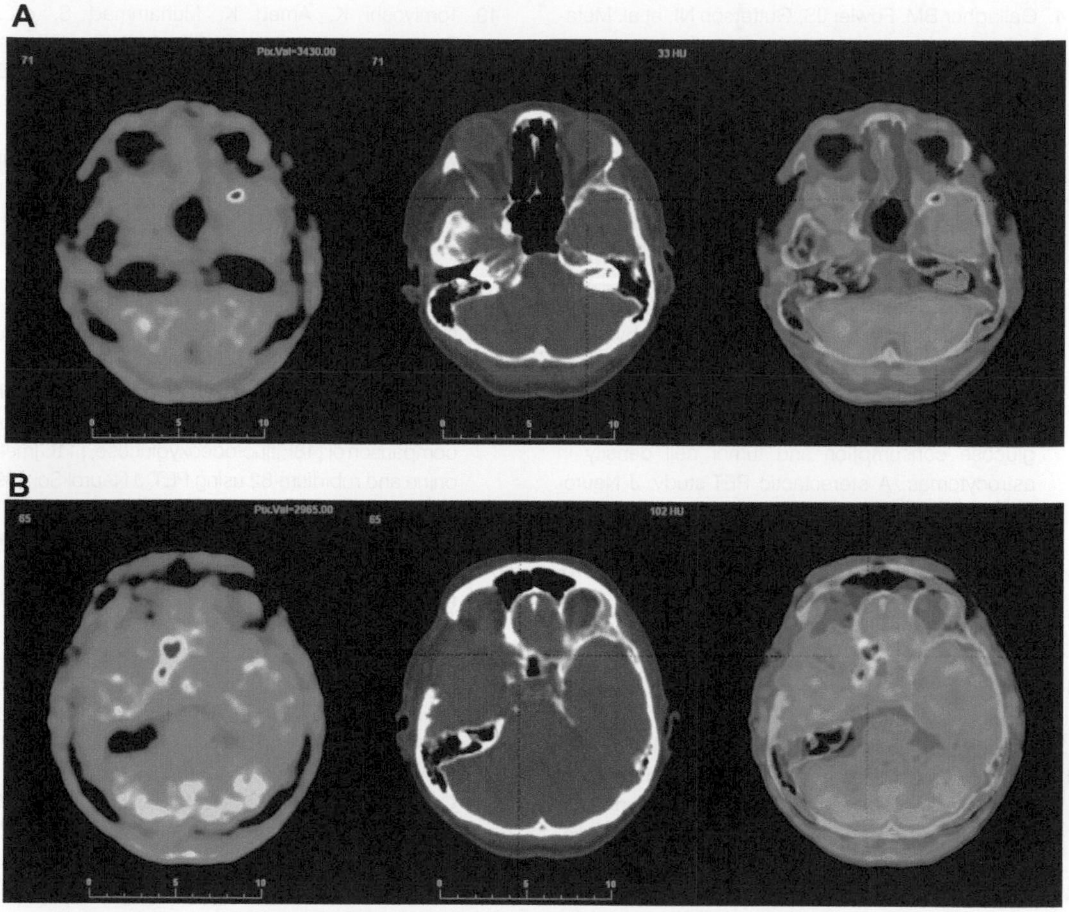

Fig. 5. A bifocal meningioma of the base of the skull. The F-TYR PET/CT showed both lesions with a high contrast, as well as the bone invasion (*A, B*).

nonresponders after one cycle of temozolomide. The same group further showed that early changes in MRGlu predicted the response only in patients with high-grade gliomas treated by temozolomide alone for recurrent disease, whereas it had no predictive value in patients with newly diagnosed disease submitted to a classic combination scheme that included radiation therapy.[97] Temozolomide also may be used in a small proportion of patients with low-grade gliomas. FET-PET performed as early as 3 months after initiating the treatment was highly predictive of the tumor volume reduction observed on MRI later on.[98] FLT, however, may prove to be the tracer of choice, as its uptake is correlated strongly with the proliferative rate of high-grade gliomas.[99] In a series of 19 patients with recurrent malignant gliomas treated by bevacizumab and irinotecan, the evolution of the FLT was correlated with the survival.[100] In fact, multivariate analysis concluded that an absence of metabolic response was among all clinical and imaging variables the strongest predictor of death.

All the available series are limited in numbers and should be considered as pilot studies. Furthermore, as pointed out by Herholz in a recent editorial, progress in brain tumor treatment has been painfully slow, and the prognosis of high-grade gliomas remains awfully dire.[101] As an imaging method, PET can only contribute as much as effective treatments are available.

REFERENCES

1. American Cancer Society. Cancer Facts & Figures 2009. Atlanta: American Cancer Society; 2009.
2. Louis DN, Ohgaki H, Wiestler OD, et al. The 2007 WHO classification of tumours of the central nervous system. Acta Neuropathol 2007;114:97.
3. Scarabino T, Popolizio T, Trojsi F, et al. Role of advanced MR imaging modalities in diagnosing cerebral gliomas. Radiol Med 2009;114:448.

4. Gallagher BM, Fowler JS, Gutterson NI, et al. Metabolic trapping as a principle of oradiopharmaceutical design: some factors resposible for the biodistribution of [18F] 2-deoxy-2-fluoro-D-glucose. J Nucl Med 1978;19:1154.
5. Nishioka T, Oda Y, Seino Y, et al. Distribution of the glucose transporters in human brain tumors. Cancer Res 1992;52:3972.
6. Weber G. Enzymology of cancer cells (first of two parts). N Engl J Med 1977;296:486.
7. Di Chiro G, DeLaPaz RL, Brooks RA, et al. Glucose utilization of cerebral gliomas measured by [18F] fluorodeoxyglucose and positron emission tomography. Neurology 1982;32:1323.
8. Herholz K, Pietrzyk U, Voges J, et al. Correlation of glucose consumption and tumor cell density in astrocytomas. A stereotactic PET study. J Neurosurg 1993;79:853.
9. Stockhammer F, Thomale UW, Plotkin M, et al. Association between fluorine-18-labeled fluorodeoxyglucose uptake and 1p and 19q loss of heterozygosity in World Health Organization Grade II gliomas. J Neurosurg 2007;106:633.
10. Dancey JE, Curiel R, Purvis J. Evaluating temsirolimus activity in multiple tumors: a review of clinical trials. Semin Oncol 2009;36(Suppl 3):S46.
11. Wei LH, Su H, Hildebrandt IJ, et al. Changes in tumor metabolism as readout for Mammalian target of rapamycin kinase inhibition by rapamycin in glioblastoma. Clin Cancer Res 2008;14:3416.
12. Delbeke D, Meyerowitz C, Lapidus RL, et al. Optimal cutoff levels of F-18 fluorodeoxyglucose uptake in the differentiation of low-grade from high-grade brain tumors with PET. Radiology 1995;195:47.
13. Kim CK, Alavi JB, Alavi A, et al. New grading system of cerebral gliomas using positron emission tomography with F-18 fluorodeoxyglucose. J Neurooncol 1991;10:85.
14. Hustinx R, Smith RJ, Benard F, et al. Can the standardized uptake value characterize primary brain tumors on FDG-PET? Eur J Nucl Med 1999;26:1501.
15. Lilja A, Bergstrom K, Hartvig P, et al. Dynamic study of supratentorial gliomas with L-methyl-11C-methionine and positron emission tomography. AJNR Am J Neuroradiol 1985;6:505.
16. Vaalburg W, Coenen HH, Crouzel C, et al. Amino acids for the measurement of protein synthesis in vivo by PET. Int J Rad Appl Instrum B 1992;19:227.
17. Coenen HH, Kling P, Stocklin G. Cerebral metabolism of L-[2-18F]fluorotyrosine, a new PET tracer of protein synthesis. J Nucl Med 1989;30:1367.
18. Luxen A, Perlmutter M, Bida GT, et al. Remote, semiautomated production of 6-[18F]fluoro-L-dopa for human studies with PET. Int J Rad Appl Instrum A 1990;41:275.
19. Tomiyoshi K, Amed K, Muhammad S, et al. Synthesis of isomers of 18F-labelled amino acid radiopharmaceutical: position 2- and 3-L-18F-alpha-methyltyrosine using a separation and purification system. Nucl Med Commun 1997;18:169.
20. Wester HJ, Herz M, Weber W, et al. Synthesis and radiopharmacology of O-(2-[18F]fluoroethyl)-L-tyrosine for tumor imaging. J Nucl Med 1999;40:205.
21. Ishiwata K, Kubota K, Murakami M, et al. A comparative study on protein incorporation of L-[methyl-3H]methionine, L-[1-14C]leucine and L-2-[18F]fluorotyrosine in tumor bearing mice. Nucl Med Biol 1993;20:895.
22. Roelcke U, Radu EW, von Ammon K, et al. Alteration of blood-brain barrier in human brain tumors: comparison of [18F]fluorodeoxyglucose, [11C]methionine and rubidium-82 using PET. J Neurol Sci 1995;132:20.
23. Lahoutte T, Caveliers V, Camargo SM, et al. SPECT and PET amino acid tracer influx via system L (h4F2hc-hLAT1) and its trans-stimulation. J Nucl Med 2004;45:1591.
24. Langen KJ, Hamacher K, Weckesser M, et al. O-(2-[18F]fluoroethyl)-L-tyrosine: uptake mechanisms and clinical applications. Nucl Med Biol 2006;33:287.
25. Langen KJ, Jarosch M, Muhlensiepen H, et al. Comparison of fluorotyrosines and methionine uptake in F98 rat gliomas. Nucl Med Biol 2003;30:501.
26. Toyohara J, Waki A, Takamatsu S, et al. Basis of FLT as a cell proliferation marker: comparative uptake studies with [3H]thymidine and [3H]arabinothymidine, and cell-analysis in 22 asynchronously growing tumor cell lines. Nucl Med Biol 2002;29:281.
27. DeGrado TR, Baldwin SW, Wang S, et al. Synthesis and evaluation of 18F-labeled choline analogs as oncologic PET tracers. J Nucl Med 2001;42:1805.
28. Hara T. 18F-fluorocholine: a new oncologic PET tracer. J Nucl Med 2001;42:1815.
29. Hara T, Kosaka N, Shinoura N, et al. PET imaging of brain tumor with [methyl-11C]choline. J Nucl Med 1997;38:842.
30. Wald LL, Nelson SJ, Day MR, et al. Serial proton magnetic resonance spectroscopy imaging of glioblastoma multiforme after brachytherapy. J Neurosurg 1997;87:525.
31. Decristoforo C, Knopp R, von Guggenberg E, et al. A fully automated synthesis for the preparation of 68Ga-labelled peptides. Nucl Med Commun 2007;28:870.
32. Henze M, Schuhmacher J, Hipp P, et al. PET imaging of somatostatin receptors using [68GA]DOTA-D-Phe1-Tyr3-octreotide: first results in patients with meningiomas. J Nucl Med 2001;42:1053.

33. Kaschten B, Stevenaert A, Sadzot B, et al. Preoperative evaluation of 54 gliomas by PET with fluorine-18-fluorodeoxyglucose and/or carbon-11-methionine. J Nucl Med 1998;39:778.
34. Ogawa T, Inugami A, Hatazawa J, et al. Clinical positron emission tomography for brain tumors: comparison of fludeoxyglucose F 18 and L-methyl-11C-methionine. AJNR Am J Neuroradiol 1996;17:345.
35. Kosaka N, Tsuchida T, Uematsu H, et al. 18F-FDG PET of common enhancing malignant brain tumors. AJR Am J Roentgenol 2008;190:W365.
36. Kitajima K, Nakamoto Y, Okizuka H, et al. Accuracy of whole-body FDG-PET/CT for detecting brain metastases from non-central nervous system tumors. Ann Nucl Med 2008;22:595.
37. Posther KE, McCall LM, Harpole DH Jr, et al. Yield of brain 18F-FDG PET in evaluating patients with potentially operable nonsmall cell lung cancer. J Nucl Med 2006;47:1607.
38. Ogawa T, Shishido F, Kanno I, et al. Cerebral glioma: evaluation with methionine PET. Radiology 1993;186:45.
39. Braun V, Dempf S, Weller R, et al. Cranial neuronavigation with direct integration of 11Cmethionine positron emission tomography (PET) data – results of a pilot study in 32 surgical cases. Acta Neurochir (Wien) 2002;144:777.
40. Herholz K, Holzer T, Bauer B, et al. 11C-methionine PET for differential diagnosis of low-grade gliomas. Neurology 1998;50:1316.
41. Kracht LW, Miletic H, Busch S, et al. Delineation of brain tumor extent with [11C]L-methionine positron emission tomography: local comparison with stereotactic histopathology. Clin Cancer Res 2004;10:7163.
42. Yamane T, Sakamoto S, Senda M. Clinical impact of (11C)-methionine PET on expected management of patients with brain neoplasm. Eur J Nucl Med Mol Imaging 2010;37:685–90.
43. Galldiks N, Kracht LW, Berthold F, et al. [11C]-L-methionine positron emission tomography in the management of children and young adults with brain tumors. J Neurooncol 2010;96:231.
44. Pauleit D, Floeth F, Hamacher K, et al. O-(2-[18F]fluoroethyl)-L-tyrosine PET combined with MRI improves the diagnostic assessment of cerebral gliomas. Brain 2005;128:678.
45. Pauleit D, Stoffels G, Bachofner A, et al. Comparison of 18F-FET and 18F-FDG PET in brain tumors. Nucl Med Biol 2009;36:779.
46. Floeth FW, Pauleit D, Sabel M, et al. 18F-FET PET differentiation of ring-enhancing brain lesions. J Nucl Med 2006;47:776.
47. Becherer A, Karanikas G, Szabo M, et al. Brain tumour imaging with PET: a comparison between [18F]fluorodopa and [11C]methionine. Eur J Nucl Med Mol Imaging 2003;30:1561.
48. Chen W, Silverman DH, Delaloye S, et al. 18F-FDOPA PET imaging of brain tumors: comparison study with 18F-FDG PET and evaluation of diagnostic accuracy. J Nucl Med 2006;47:904.
49. De Witte O, Goldberg I, Wikler D, et al. Positron emission tomography with injection of methionine as a prognostic factor in glioma. J Neurosurg 2001;95:746.
50. Kameyama M, Shirane R, Itoh J, et al. The accumulation of 11C-methionine in cerebral glioma patients studied with PET. Acta Neurochir (Wien) 1990;104:8.
51. Kato T, Shinoda J, Nakayama N, et al. Metabolic assessment of gliomas using 11C-methionine, [18F] fluorodeoxyglucose, and 11C-choline positron-emission tomography. AJNR Am J Neuroradiol 2008;29:1176.
52. Ceyssens S, Van Laere K, de Groot T, et al. [11C]methionine PET, histopathology, and survival in primary brain tumors and recurrence. AJNR Am J Neuroradiol 2006;27:1432.
53. Moulin-Romsee G, D'Hondt E, de Groot T, et al. Non-invasive grading of brain tumours using dynamic amino acid PET imaging: does it work for 11C-methionine? Eur J Nucl Med Mol Imaging 2007;34:2082.
54. Stockhammer F, Plotkin M, Amthauer H, et al. Correlation of F-18-fluoro-ethyl-tyrosin uptake with vascular and cell density in non-contrast-enhancing gliomas. J Neurooncol 2008;88:205.
55. Popperl G, Kreth FW, Mehrkens JH, et al. FET PET for the evaluation of untreated gliomas: correlation of FET uptake and uptake kinetics with tumour grading. Eur J Nucl Med Mol Imaging 2007;34:1933.
56. Alavi JB, Alavi A, Chawluk J, et al. Positron emission tomography in patients with glioma. A predictor of prognosis. Cancer 1988;62:1074.
57. Patronas NJ, Brooks RA, DeLaPaz RL, et al. Glycolytic rate (PET) and contrast enhancement (CT) in human cerebral gliomas. AJNR Am J Neuroradiol 1983;4:533.
58. De Witte O, Levivier M, Violon P, et al. Prognostic value positron emission tomography with [18F]fluoro-2-deoxy-D-glucose in the low-grade glioma. Neurosurgery 1996;39:470.
59. Kruer MC, Kaplan AM, Etzl MM Jr, et al. The value of positron emission tomography and proliferation index in predicting progression in low-grade astrocytomas of childhood. J Neurooncol 2009;95:239.
60. Floeth FW, Pauleit D, Sabel M, et al. Prognostic value of O-(2-18F-fluoroethyl)-L-tyrosine PET and MRI in low-grade glioma. J Nucl Med 2007;48:519.
61. Hanson MW, Glantz MJ, Hoffman JM, et al. FDG-PET in the selection of brain lesions for biopsy. J Comput Assist Tomogr 1991;15:796.

62. Pirotte B, Goldman S, Bidaut LM, et al. Use of positron emission tomography (PET) in stereotactic conditions for brain biopsy. Acta Neurochir (Wien) 1995;134:79.
63. Pirotte B, Goldman S, Massager N, et al. Comparison of 18F-FDG and 11C-methionine for PET-guided stereotactic brain biopsy of gliomas. J Nucl Med 2004;45:1293.
64. Pirotte BJ, Lubansu A, Massager N, et al. Results of positron emission tomography guidance and reassessment of the utility of and indications for stereotactic biopsy in children with infiltrative brainstem tumors. J Neurosurg 2007;107:392.
65. Maier H, Ofner D, Hittmair A, et al. Classic, atypical, and anaplastic meningioma: three histopathological subtypes of clinical relevance. J Neurosurg 1992;77:616.
66. Cremerius U, Bares R, Weis J, et al. Fasting improves discrimination of grade 1 and atypical or malignant meningioma in FDG-PET. J Nucl Med 1997;38:26.
67. Di Chiro G, Hatazawa J, Katz DA, et al. Glucose utilization by intracranial meningiomas as an index of tumor aggressivity and probability of recurrence: a PET study. Radiology 1987;164:521.
68. Lee JW, Kang KW, Park SH, et al. 18F-FDG PET in the assessment of tumor grade and prediction of tumor recurrence in intracranial meningioma. Eur J Nucl Med Mol Imaging 2009;36:1574.
69. Giovacchini G, Fallanca F, Landoni C, et al. C-11 choline versus F-18 fluorodeoxyglucose for imaging meningiomas: an initial experience. Clin Nucl Med 2009;34:7.
70. Giglio P, Gilbert MR. Cerebral radiation necrosis. Neurologist 2003;9:180.
71. Plowman PN. Stereotactic radiosurgery. VIII. The classification of postradiation reactions. Br J Neurosurg 1999;13:256.
72. Patronas NJ, Di Chiro G, Brooks RA, et al. Work in progress: [18F] fluorodeoxyglucose and positron emission tomography in the evaluation of radiation necrosis of the brain. Radiology 1982; 144:885.
73. Chao ST, Suh JH, Raja S, et al. The sensitivity and specificity of FDG PET in distinguishing recurrent brain tumor from radionecrosis in patients treated with stereotactic radiosurgery. Int J Cancer 2001; 96:191.
74. Gomez-Rio M, Rodriguez-Fernandez A, Ramos-Font C, et al. Diagnostic accuracy of 201Thallium-SPECT and 18F-FDG-PET in the clinical assessment of glioma recurrence. Eur J Nucl Med Mol Imaging 2008;35:966.
75. Kahn D, Follott KA, Bushnell DL, et al. Diagnosis of recurrent brain tumor: value of 201Tl SPECT vs 18F-fluorodeoxyglucose PET. AJR Am J Roentgenol 1994;163:1459.
76. Alexiou GA, Tsiouris S, Kyritsis AP, et al. Glioma recurrence versus radiation necrosis: accuracy of current imaging modalities. J Neurooncol 2009;95:1.
77. Terakawa Y, Tsuyuguchi N, Iwai Y, et al. Diagnostic accuracy of 11C-methionine PET for differentiation of recurrent brain tumors from radiation necrosis after radiotherapy. J Nucl Med 2008;49:694.
78. Van Laere K, Ceyssens S, Van Calenbergh F, et al. Direct comparison of 18F-FDG and 11C-methionine PET in suspected recurrence of glioma: sensitivity, inter-observer variability and prognostic value. Eur J Nucl Med Mol Imaging 2005;32:39.
79. Mehrkens JH, Popperl G, Rachinger W, et al. The positive predictive value of O-(2-[18F]fluoroethyl)-L-tyrosine (FET) PET in the diagnosis of a glioma recurrence after multimodal treatment. J Neurooncol 2008;88:27.
80. Rachinger W, Goetz C, Popperl G, et al. Positron emission tomography with O-(2-[18F]fluoroethyl)-l-tyrosine versus magnetic resonance imaging in the diagnosis of recurrent gliomas. Neurosurgery 2005;57:505.
81. Yamamoto Y, Wong TZ, Turkington TG, et al. 3′-Deoxy-3′-[F18]fluorothymidine positron emission tomography in patients with recurrent glioblastoma multiforme: comparison with Gd-DTPA enhanced magnetic resonance imaging. Mol Imaging Biol 2006;8:340.
82. Maher EA, McKee A. Neoplasms of the central nervous system. In: Skarin AT, editor. Atlas of diagnostic oncology. London: Elsevier Science Limited; 2003. p. 403–15.
83. Francavilla TL, Miletich RS, Di Chiro G, et al. Positron emission tomography in the detection of malignant degeneration of low-grade gliomas. Neurosurgery 1989;24:1.
84. Ullrich RT, Kracht L, Brunn A, et al. Methyl-L-11C-methionine PET as a diagnostic marker for malignant progression in patients with glioma. J Nucl Med 2009;50:1962.
85. Piroth MD, Pinkawa M, Holy R, et al. Integrated-boost IMRT or 3-D-CRT using FET-PET based auto-contoured target volume delineation for glioblastoma multiforme—a dosimetric comparison. Radiat Oncol 2009;4:57.
86. Douglas JG, Stelzer KJ, Mankoff DA, et al. [F18]-fluorodeoxyglucose positron emission tomography for targeting radiation dose escalation for patients with glioblastoma multiforme: clinical outcomes and patterns of failure. Int J Radiat Oncol Biol Phys 2006;64:886.
87. Tralins KS, Douglas JG, Stelzer KJ, et al. Volumetric analysis of 18F-FDG PET in glioblastoma multiforme: prognostic information and possible role in definition of target volumes in radiation dose escalation. J Nucl Med 2002;43:1667.

88. Grosu AL, Weber WA, Riedel E, et al. L-(methyl-11C) methionine positron emission tomography for target delineation in resected high-grade gliomas before radiotherapy. Int J Radiat Oncol Biol Phys 2005;63:64.
89. Mahasittiwat P, Mizoe JE, Hasegawa A, et al. l-[METHYL-11C] methionine positron emission tomography for target delineation in malignant gliomas: impact on results of carbon ion radiotherapy. Int J Radiat Oncol Biol Phys 2008;70:515.
90. Weber DC, Zilli T, Buchegger F, et al. [18F]Fluoroethyltyrosine- positron emission tomography-guided radiotherapy for high-grade glioma. Radiat Oncol 2008;3:44.
91. Gehler B, Paulsen F, Oksuz MO, et al. [68Ga]-DOTATOC-PET/CT for meningioma IMRT treatment planning. Radiat Oncol 2009;4:56.
92. Milker-Zabel S, Zabel-du Bois A, Henze M, et al. Improved target volume definition for fractionated stereotactic radiotherapy in patients with intracranial meningiomas by correlation of CT, MRI, and [68Ga]-DOTATOC-PET. Int J Radiat Oncol Biol Phys 2006;65:222.
93. Rutten I, Cabay JE, Withofs N, et al. PET/CT of skull base meningiomas using 2-18F-fluoro-L-tyrosine: initial report. J Nucl Med 2007;48:720.
94. Grosu AL, Weber WA, Astner ST, et al. 11C-methionine PET improves the target volume delineation of meningiomas treated with stereotactic fractionated radiotherapy. Int J Radiat Oncol Biol Phys 2006;66:339.
95. Stupp R, Mason WP, van den Bent MJ, et al. Radiotherapy plus concomitant and adjuvant temozolomide for glioblastoma. N Engl J Med 2005;352:987.
96. Brock CS, Young H, O'Reilly SM, et al. Early evaluation of tumour metabolic response using [18F]fluorodeoxyglucose and positron emission tomography: a pilot study following the phase II chemotherapy schedule for temozolomide in recurrent high-grade gliomas. Br J Cancer 2000;82:608.
97. Charnley N, West CM, Barnett CM, et al. Early change in glucose metabolic rate measured using FDG-PET in patients with high-grade glioma predicts response to temozolomide but not temozolomide plus radiotherapy. Int J Radiat Oncol Biol Phys 2006;66:331.
98. Wyss M, Hofer S, Bruehlmeier M, et al. Early metabolic responses in temozolomide treated low-grade glioma patients. J Neurooncol 2009;95:87.
99. Backes H, Ullrich R, Neumaier B, et al. Noninvasive quantification of 18F-FLT human brain PET for the assessment of tumour proliferation in patients with high-grade glioma. Eur J Nucl Med Mol Imaging 2009;36:1960–7.
100. Chen W, Delaloye S, Silverman DH, et al. Predicting treatment response of malignant gliomas to bevacizumab and irinotecan by imaging proliferation with [18F] fluorothymidine positron emission tomography: a pilot study. J Clin Oncol 2007;25:4714.
101. Herholz K. Amino acid PET and clinical management of glioma patients. Eur J Nucl Med Mol Imaging 2010;37:683–4.

PET Imaging for Traumatic Brain Injury

Jacob G. Dubroff, MD, PhD, Andrew B. Newberg, MD*

KEYWORDS

- Traumatic brain injury • Diffuse axonal injury
- PET • Fluorodeoxyglucose

With over 1.5 million annual incidences resulting in an estimated 50,000 deaths, 300,000 hospitalizations, 80,000 to 90,000 long-term disabled individuals and estimated costs at greater than $60 billion, traumatic brain injury (TBI) represents a major health problem in the United States.[1–3] Neuroimaging is critical for timely, accurate diagnosis and optimal management of the TBI patient. Although plain radiographs, magnetic resonance imaging (MRI), single photon emission computed tomography (SPECT) and PET all have been employed, computed tomography (CT) represents the principal imaging modality for TBI. This likely will and should continue because of CT's exceptional ability to demonstrate skull fractures, epidural hematomas, subdural hematomas, and other acute pathologies associated with TBI that require expedited management decisions.[3–7]

Once outside of the critical management window, the additional afore-mentioned neuroimaging modalities may be of value. Because the arsenal remains limited to treat TBI and the understanding of TBI pathophysiology also remains primitive, in vivo central nervous system (CNS) imaging advances will continue to shape patient management. Specifically, because the basis of PET imaging is underlying cellular molecular biologic change, it has the potential to provide unique insights into this disease and its treatment. This article will examine the body of PET imaging focused upon traumatic brain injury and contemplate PET's role in future experimental and, possibly, clinical practice.

FLUORODEOXYGLUCOSE AND PET

The most prominent contemporary role in medicine of PET is revealing the locations of glucose hypermetabolism indicative of neoplastic disease.[8,9] By superimposing function on anatomy, PET/CT has shown superiority compared with PET alone in cancer mapping, and that is why combination machines are rapidly replacing PET-only ones.[9–14] Before the existence, availability, and popularity of functional MRI (fMRI), it is important to note that PET first was used to visualize in vivo human brain function.[15,16]

The radiotracer ^{18}F-fluorodeoxyglucose (^{18}F-FDG) usually is inferred when PET imaging is mentioned. It is a glucose analog, and, within mitochondria, metabolized by hexokinase to ^{18}F-FDG-6-phosphate rather than 2-deoxy-D-glucose, whereby it becomes trapped and continues to emit a positron.[17] Not surprisingly, the more severe the head injury, the more likely a reduction in brain glucose metabolism will be detected.[18,19] As in the case of stroke, Alzheimer's-type dementia and Pick's disease, FDG-PET demonstration of focal metabolic defects often correlate with specific functional deficits endured by TBI patients (**Fig. 1**).

FDG-PET also can detect abnormalities in TBI patients when they are absent on MRI and CT.[20–23] Some studies have revealed that as much as 42% of PET abnormalities were not associated with any lesions observed on anatomic images.[24,25] Lesions such as cortical contusions, intracranial hematomas, and subsequent encephalomalacias

Division of Nuclear Medicine, Department of Radiology, Hospital of the University of Pennsylvania, Room 110, Donner Building, Philadelphia, PA 19104, USA
* Corresponding author.
E-mail address: andrew.newberg@uphs.upenn.edu

PET Clin 5 (2010) 199–207
doi:10.1016/j.cpet.2010.01.002

usually are confined to the site of injury, while subdural and epidural hematomas often cause widespread hypometabolism and even may affect the contralateral hemisphere.[24,25] Diffuse axonal injury has been found to cause diffuse cortical hypometabolism and a marked decrease in parieto–occipital cortical metabolism.[24–26] An example of this finding is illustrated in **Fig. 2**. Lupi and colleagues also noted a pattern of relatively increased metabolism of the cerebellar vermis in 54 of 57 TBI patients.[27] **Fig. 3** demonstrates such an example.

FDG-PET also has been of great value in revealing seizure foci.[28–32] Specifically, epileptogenic foci are thought to be hypometabolic during interictal status and reflected by a decrease in radiotracer distribution.[30,32] FDG-PET therefore, has been used to identify such regions in mesial temporal lobe epilepsy and types of focal cortical dysplasias.[29,31] Ferguson recently published a retrospective analysis of TBI patients and their respective risk of developing post-traumatic encephalopathy (PTE) and found an incremental risk corresponding to severity of injury.[33] Within 3 years after being discharged, patients with mild, moderate, and severe TBIs had an incidence of developing epilepsy of 4.4, 7.6, and 13.6 per 100 persons, respectively.[33] FDG-PET even has been used to help guide whether a combat pilot could return to duty after a TBI.[34]

PET: ^{15}O

Although PET imaging usually is assumed to map glucose metabolism, there are several other tracers that have been employed to study TBI. Even though it requires a cyclotron facility on premises because of its short half-life, positron-labeled oxygen (^{15}O water) has been used successfully in several PET TBI studies.[35–46] Because of its short 2-minute half-life, any ^{15}O injection and consequent imaging are technically demanding and also require some time for preparation. This complexity is amplified in the clinical setting of a TBI patient, especially one in critical status, making it very impractical.

Despite the challenge of using such a short-lived isotope, ^{15}O has been used to examine the role of hypoxia in TBI because of the ischemic cell damage that occurs in 90% of these patients. This ischemia likely is mediated by the release of various toxins in response to the molecular events associated with brain injury, which, in turn, also may lead to an ischemia–reperfusion injury.[47,48]

Such ^{15}O studies have demonstrated increased oxygen extraction fraction in regions of brain with reduced cerebral blood flow[40,45]; however, such oxygen delivery within hypoxic brain may not achieve normal diffusion rates.[41] These studies also have attempted to establish an ischemic burden of injury in the TBI patient.[37,38] For example, Cunningham and colleagues[38] demonstrated that although cerebral oxygen use in the TBI patient is comparable with that observed in stroke patients, cerebral blood flow thresholds are inherently different between the two patient populations. The heterogeneity of TBIs only further complicates the comprehension of its pathophysiology.

Although ^{15}O PET imaging may offer a global map of brain oxygenation in the traumatic brain injured patient, it represents but a small period of time. Therefore, ^{15}O PET imaging also has been correlated with more invasive, localized, and dynamic measurements of brain oxygen content,

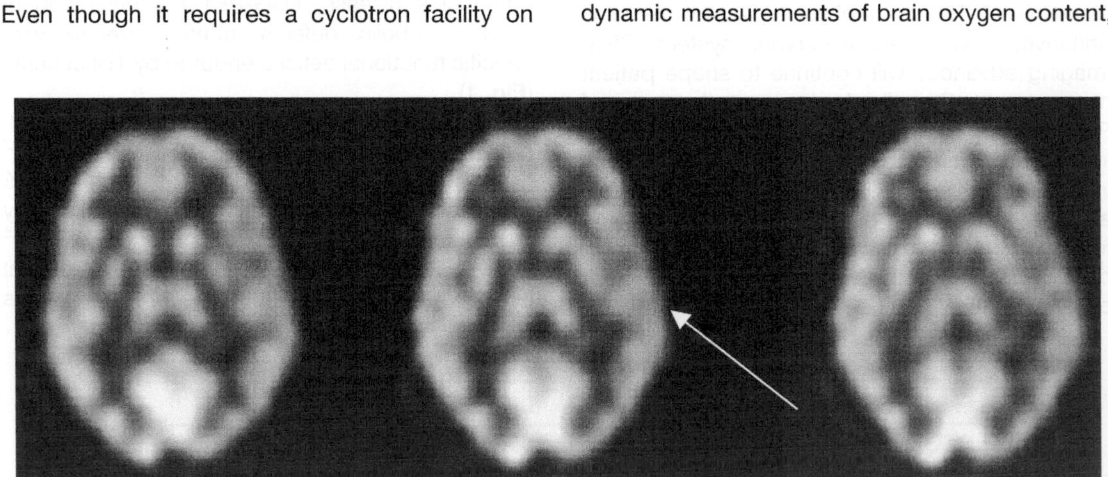

Fig. 1. FDG-PET scan of a 43-year old woman who suffered a head injury 2 years before this study and now has cognitive and memory dysfunction and language problems. This scan demonstrates hypometabolism of the entire left hemisphere *(arrow)* relative to the right. *Abbreviation:* FDG-PET, fluorodeoxyglucose–PET.

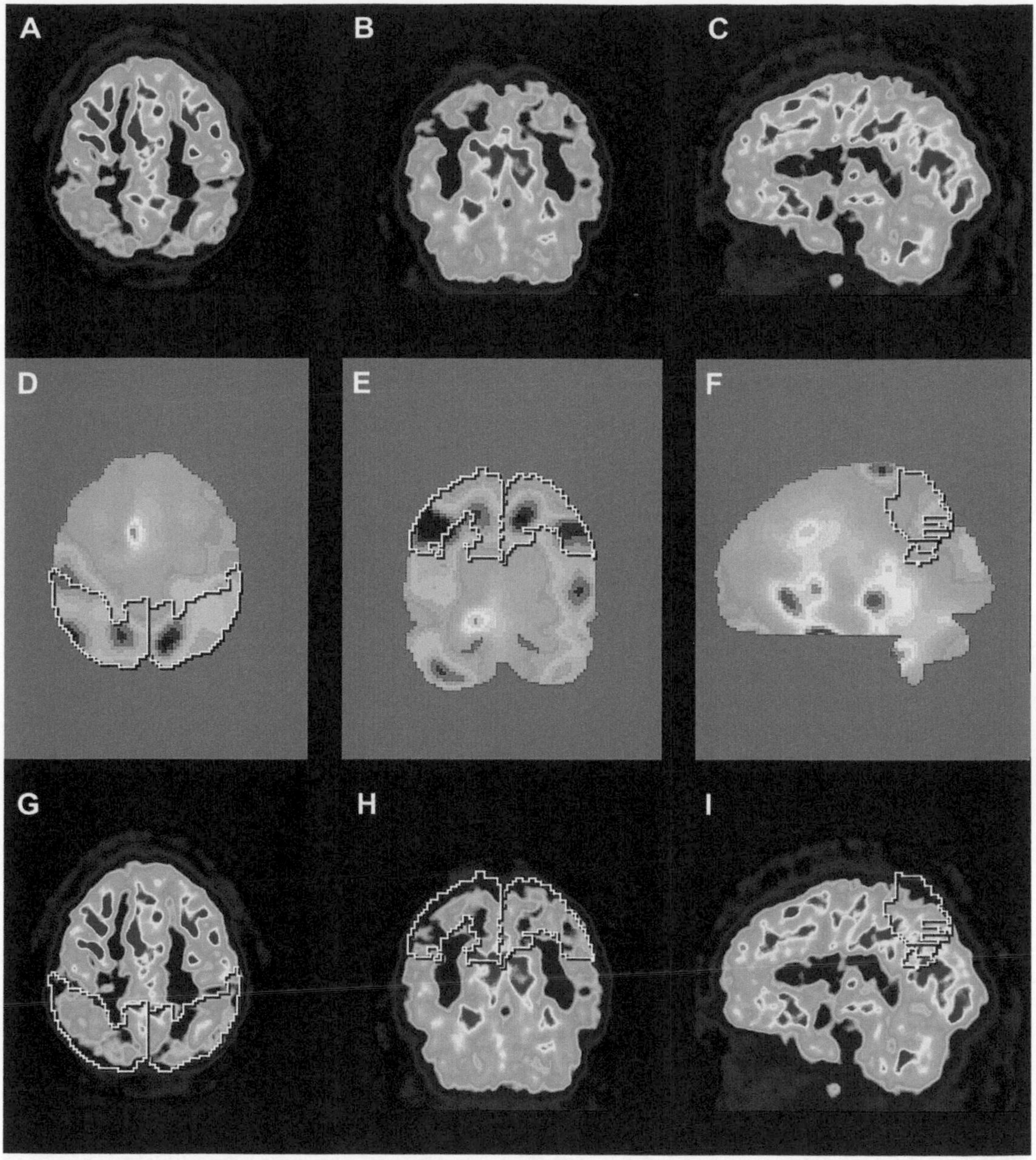

Fig. 2. FDG-PET scan of a 31-year-old man with diffuse axonal injury demonstrating bilateral parietal hypometabolism. The PET images used for interpretation are shown in row 1 in the axial *(A)*, coronal *(B)*, and sagittal *(C)* planes. Row 2 demonstrates bilateral parietal regions of interest (ROI) determined using Siemens Scenium quantification software in the axial *(D)*, coronal *(E)*, and sagittal *(F)* planes. Row 3 shows the same bilateral ROI superimposed on the original FDG-PET images in the axial *(G)*, coronal *(H)*, and sagittal *(I)* planes.

including oxygen saturation of jugular blood[36] and measurements obtained with in vivo microdialysis catheters.[35,39,42,46] PET imaging, however, did not correlate well with the lactate to pyruvate ratio, which should be greater than 1 under aerobic conditions,[42,46] suggesting a state of metabolic dysfunction unrelated to ischemia. Such future studies correlating PET imaging with other biomarkers will be of critical importance in placing PET imaging within the proper clinical context.

PET: COREGISTRATION WITH MRI

Unfortunately, most brain glucose metabolism defects after TBI are fairly uniform across varying

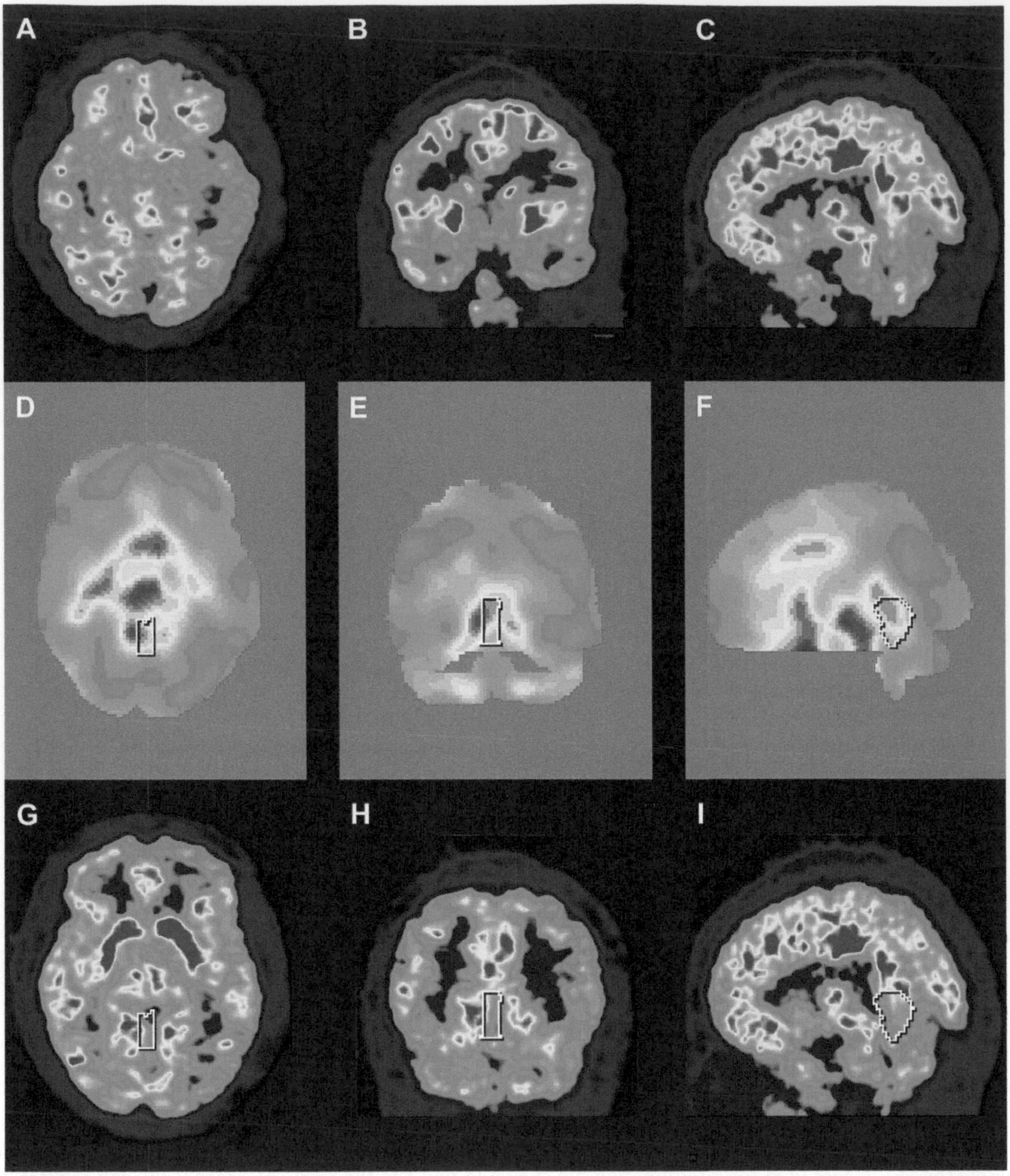

Fig. 3. FDG-PET brain scan of a 19-year-old man with an intracranial injury. Although there are no metabolic defects obvious to even the seasoned interpreter in the clinical study seen in row 1 in the axial *(A)*, coronal *(B)*, and sagittal *(C)* planes, quantification technique reveals increased metabolism in the vermis and in row 2 in the axial *(D)*, coronal *(E)*, and sagittal *(F)* planes. ROI determined by quantification software again are superimposed on the original scan in row 3 in the axial *(G)*, coronal *(H)*, and sagittal *(I)* planes.

TBI subtypes and severities.[49] Yet, there is evidence that FDG-PET is superior to neuropsychological assessment in predicting cognitive decline of the TBI patient.[25] In patients whose cognitive decline could have multiple etiologies (eg, TBI versus Alzheimer disease versus vascular dementia), the FDG-PET pattern can be distinct for each condition. The major limitation of FDG-PET is that it cannot distinguish between functional abnormalities specifically related to structural damage and those functional abnormalities that are not associated with clear structural damage.[50] Thus, it is essential that PET images be compared with corresponding anatomic images.

Because the brain is a rigid body, FDG-PET and MRI can be coregistered readily using commercially available software. Fusion of FDG-PET and MRI studies is likely to continue to gain popularity. For example, Salamon and colleagues[31] demonstrated that coregistration of FDG-PET with MRI improved cortical dysplasia lesion detection in surgical epilepsy patients. An example of FDG-PET and MRI image coregistration is shown in **Fig. 4**.

PET QUANTIFICATION TECHNIQUES

The semiquantitative standard uptake value (SUV) usually is employed in FDG-PET clinical practice when longitudinally documenting tumor activity.[51] The maximum SUV of given neoplastic lesion has prognostic value in charting the behavior of numerous solid tumors including lymphomas (Hodgkin lymphoma and non-Hodgkin lymphoma [NHL]) as well as bladder, breast, non-small cell lung, esophageal, head and neck, colorectal, ovarian and cervical cancers.[52–64] Specifically, the idea of using semi-quantitative PET analysis to determine therapeutic response in oncology is gaining momentum.[65,66]

Quantification of FDG-PET in brain studies has been performed using several arithmetic methods including region of interest (ROI) and statistical parametric mapping.[67–69] Practically, its use in temporal lobe epilepsy may be of greatest current value.[29] The major PET machine manufacturers, including Siemens (Scenium; Hoffman Estates, IL, USA), Philips (NeuroQ; Andover, MD, USA) and General Electric (Cortex ID; Piscataway, NJ, USA), offer brain quantification software, and there a growing number of free online resources also. The challenge of using FDG-PET in the subacute and chronic stages of TBI is the heterogeneity of presentations. Some studies, however, have used such a systematic approach, including Lupi and colleagues, who found that hypermetabolism of the cerebellar vermis is a highly consistent finding in the TBI patient.[27] An example of hypermetabolism in the vermis is shown in **Fig. 3**. Note that purely qualitative interpretation of the PET images likely would not detect such a finding. Therefore, future investigations using serial studies in individual patients examining change over time and comparison to a standardized, age-normalized PET brain atlas could be fruitful in revealing abnormalities and validating interventions. For example, Krauss and colleagues examined the effect of amantadine treatment on cerebral glucose patterns in chronic TBI patients and found this therapy increased left prefrontal cortex metabolism, which positively correlated with executive domain scores.[70]

NOVEL RADIONUCLIDES

Part of the unique promise of PET lays in the development of new compounds that have the potential to reveal specific molecular pathways as is the case for FDG and glycolysis. Although complicated chemistry and radiochemistry often prove to be formidable hurdles, and an on-premises cyclotron facility is required, the knowledge gained through use of PET in TBI patients is well worth the challenge.

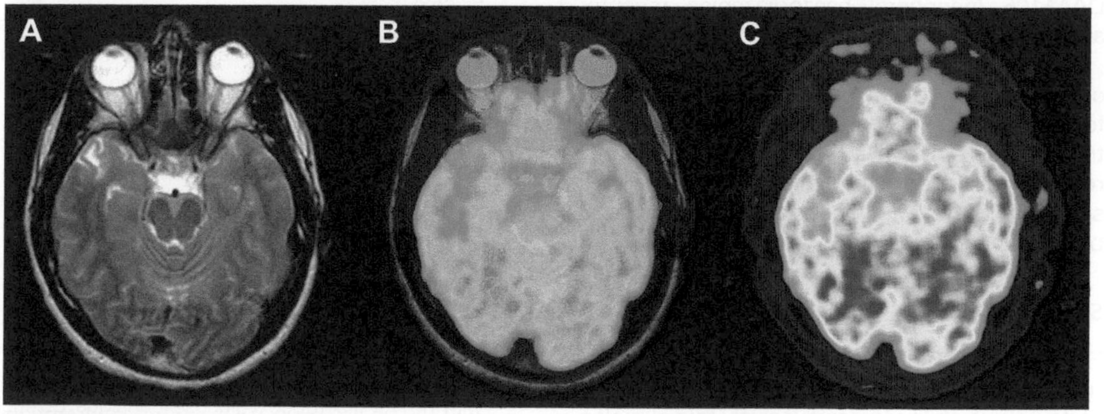

Fig. 4. FDG-PET scan coregistered with a T2 magnetic resonance imaging (MRI) scan of a 37-year-old man with a history of traumatic brain injury and intractable seizures. Included in **Fig. 3** are *(A)* MRI T2 only, *(B)* FDG-PET coregistered with MRI-T2, and *(C)* FDG-PET only. Note the hyperintense, cystic lesion in the anterior right temporal horn a region of hypometabolism just posterior. This lesion is thought to be low-grade glioma based on its conventional MR appearance as well as MR spectroscopy. As the indication for surgical excision of low-grade gliomas remains unclear, the FDG-PET helped to implicate this lesion of the epileptic focus amenable to surgical excision.

Despite the impracticality of ^{15}O as discussed earlier, there are existing agents that demonstrate a signal increase in locations of compromised oxygen, including F-18 EF5, F-18 F-MISO, and F-18 FAZA. All of these compounds are fluorinated and thus have 110-minute half-lives, making them more practical imaging compound candidates. These fluorinated azole compounds reveal hypoxic yet salvageable cells by binding irreversibly to intracellular macromolecules in low-oxygen environments.[71] F-MISO has been used successfully to demonstrate poststroke salvageable pneumbra in an animal model,[71–73] and, more recently, shown to be indicative of vasospasm in the post-subarachnoid hemorrhage patient.[74]

The incidence of Alzheimer dementia is increasing as a growing percentage of the US population ages. This increase in Alzheimer dementia has, in turn, stimulated interested in establishing a PET marker for abeta amyloid plaques.[75–78] Interestingly, greater amounts amyloid soluble in CSF have been correlated with improved outcome in severe TBI, suggesting an important role of beta amyloid in neuronal plasticity.[79]

There is also increasing interest in the spectrum of traumatic brain injury endured by athletes who develop early cognitive decline.[80] Postmortem examination, however, often reveals tau-immunoreactive neurofibrillary tangles, not beta amyloid plaques.[81] In vivo differentiation examining tau versus amyloid using PET imaging could help unravel the pathophysiology and time course of these dementias, but no PET tau imaging agent is currently available.

Additional PET tracers and molecular targets, including Co55-calcium, C11-flumazenil (GABA-A, gamma amino butyric acid, receptor), C11-DAA1106 (peripheral benzodiazepine receptor) also have shown great promise.[23,82–85]

It is also important to note that PET tracers continue to be developed, and their application to TBI may only be a matter of time. Despite the trend in PET/CT availability for oncology, it often remains challenging to obtain an FDG-PET brain scan for TBI patients, and it often is not covered by insurance.

SUMMARY

FDG and ^{15}O PET imaging already have offered unique and important insights into TBI. Because of its unique ability to noninvasively reveal molecular processes, the use of PET imaging will continue to grow despite its challenging technical aspects. This should directly improve understanding of TBI pathophysiology and lead to novel interventions.

REFERENCES

1. Rutland-Brown W, Langlois JA, Thomas KE, et al. Incidence of traumatic brain injury in the United States, 2003. J Head Trauma Rehabil 2006;21:544.
2. Sherer M, Stouter J, Hart T, et al. Computed tomography findings and early cognitive outcome after traumatic brain injury. Brain Inj 2006;20:997.
3. Stein SC, Burnett MG, Glick HA. Indications for CT scanning in mild traumatic brain injury: a cost-effectiveness study. J Trauma 2006;61:558.
4. Haydel MJ, Preston CA, Mills TJ, et al. Indications for computed tomography in patients with minor head injury. N Engl J Med 2000;343:100.
5. Orrison WW, Gentry LR, Stimac GK, et al. Blinded comparison of cranial CT and MR in closed head injury evaluation. AJNR Am J Neuroradiol 1994;15:351.
6. Smith JS, Chang EF, Rosenthal G, et al. The role of early follow-up computed tomography imaging in the management of traumatic brain injury patients with intracranial hemorrhage. J Trauma 2007;63:75.
7. Vilke GM, Chan TC, Guss DA. Use of a complete neurological examination to screen for significant intracranial abnormalities in minor head injury. Am J Emerg Med 2000;18:159.
8. Podoloff DA, Macapinlac HA. PET and PET/CT in management of the lymphomas. Radiol Clin North Am 2007;45:689.
9. Wynants J, Stroobants S, Dooms C, et al. Staging of lung cancer. Radiol Clin North Am 2007;45:609.
10. Antoch G, Stattaus J, Nemat AT, et al. Nonsmall cell lung cancer: dual-modality PET/CT in preoperative staging. Radiology 2003;229:526.
11. Bar-Shalom R, Guralnik L, Tsalic M, et al. The additional value of PET/CT over PET in FDG imaging of oesophageal cancer. Eur J Nucl Med Mol Imaging 2005;32:918.
12. Bar-Shalom R, Yefremov N, Guralnik L, et al. Clinical performance of PET/CT in evaluation of cancer: additional value for diagnostic imaging and patient management. J Nucl Med 2003;44:1200.
13. Kagna O, Solomonov A, Keidar Z, et al. The value of FDG-PET/CT in assessing single pulmonary nodules in patients at high risk of lung cancer. Eur J Nucl Med Mol Imaging 2009;36:997.
14. Schoder H, Yeung HW, Gonen M, et al. Head and neck cancer: clinical usefulness and accuracy of PET/CT image fusion. Radiology 2004;231:65.
15. Greenberg JH, Reivich M, Alavi A, et al. Metabolic mapping of functional activity in human subjects with the [18F]fluorodeoxyglucose technique. Science 1981;212:678.
16. Reivich M, Kuhl D, Wolf A, et al. The [18F]fluorodeoxyglucose method for the measurement of local cerebral glucose utilization in man. Circ Res 1979;44:127.

17. Alavi A, Dann R, Chawluk J, et al. Positron emission tomography imaging of regional cerebral glucose metabolism. Semin Nucl Med 1986;16:2.
18. Bergsneider M, Hovda DA, Lee SM, et al. Dissociation of cerebral glucose metabolism and level of consciousness during the period of metabolic depression following human traumatic brain injury. J Neurotrauma 2000;17:389.
19. Hattori N, Huang SC, Wu HM, et al. Correlation of regional metabolic rates of glucose with glasgow coma scale after traumatic brain injury. J Nucl Med 2003;44:1709.
20. Fontaine A, Azouvi P, Remy P, et al. Functional anatomy of neuropsychological deficits after severe traumatic brain injury. Neurology 1999;53:1963.
21. Nakamizo A, Inamura T, Amano T, et al. Decreased thalamic metabolism without thalamic magnetic resonance imaging abnormalities following shearing injury to the substantia nigra. J Clin Neurosci 2002;9:685.
22. Nakayama N, Okumura A, Shinoda J, et al. Relationship between regional cerebral metabolism and consciousness disturbance in traumatic diffuse brain injury without large focal lesions: an FDG-PET study with statistical parametric mapping analysis. J Neurol Neurosurg Psychiatr 2006;77:856.
23. Shiga T, Ikoma K, Katoh C, et al. Loss of neuronal integrity: a cause of hypometabolism in patients with traumatic brain injury without MRI abnormality in the chronic stage. Eur J Nucl Med Mol Imaging 2006;33:817.
24. Alavi A, Mirot A, Newberg A, et al. Fluorine-18-FDG evaluation of crossed cerebellar diaschisis in head injury. J Nucl Med 1997;38:1717.
25. Alavi A, Newberg AB. Metabolic consequences of acute brain trauma: is there a role for PET? J Nucl Med 1996;37:1170.
26. Kato T, Nakayama N, Yasokawa Y, et al. Statistical image analysis of cerebral glucose metabolism in patients with cognitive impairment following diffuse traumatic brain injury. J Neurotrauma 2007;24:919.
27. Lupi A, Bertagnoni G, Salgarello M, et al. Cerebellar vermis relative hypermetabolism: an almost constant PET finding in an injured brain. Clin Nucl Med 2007;32:445.
28. Henry TR, Engel J Jr, Mazziotta JC. Clinical evaluation of interictal fluorine-18-fluorodeoxyglucose PET in partial epilepsy. J Nucl Med 1993;34:1892.
29. Lin TW, de Aburto MA, Dahlbom M, et al. Predicting seizure-free status for temporal lobe epilepsy patients undergoing surgery: prognostic value of quantifying maximal metabolic asymmetry extending over a specified proportion of the temporal lobe. J Nucl Med 2007;48:776.
30. Mazziotta JC, Engel J Jr. The use and impact of positron computed tomography scanning in epilepsy. Epilepsia 1984;25(Suppl 2):S86.
31. Salamon N, Kung J, Shaw SJ, et al. FDG-PET/MRI coregistration improves detection of cortical dysplasia in patients with epilepsy. Neurology 2008;71:1594.
32. Sperling MR, Gur RC, Alavi A, et al. Subcortical metabolic alterations in partial epilepsy. Epilepsia 1990;31:145.
33. Ferguson PL, Smith GM, Wannamaker BB, et al. A population-based study of risk of epilepsy after hospitalization for traumatic brain injury. Epilepsia 2009. [Epub ahead of print].
34. Grossman A, Azaria B, Carter D, et al. PET scan as an aid for the return of a head-injured aviator to flying duty. Aviat Space Environ Med 2006;77:1080.
35. Abate MG, Trivedi M, Fryer TD, et al. Early derangements in oxygen and glucose metabolism following head injury: the ischemic penumbra and pathophysiological heterogeneity. Neurocrit Care 2008;9:319.
36. Coles JP, Fryer TD, Smielewski P, et al. Incidence and mechanisms of cerebral ischemia in early clinical head injury. J Cereb Blood Flow Metab 2004;24:202.
37. Coles JP, Fryer TD, Smielewski P, et al. Defining ischemic burden after traumatic brain injury using 15O PET imaging of cerebral physiology. J Cereb Blood Flow Metab 2004;24:191.
38. Cunningham AS, Salvador R, Coles JP, et al. Physiological thresholds for irreversible tissue damage in contusional regions following traumatic brain injury. Brain 2005;128:1931.
39. Gupta AK, Hutchinson PJ, Fryer T, et al. Measurement of brain tissue oxygenation performed using positron emission tomography scanning to validate a novel monitoring method. J Neurosurg 2002;96:263.
40. Johnston AJ, Steiner LA, Coles JP, et al. Effect of cerebral perfusion pressure augmentation on regional oxygenation and metabolism after head injury. Crit Care Med 2005;33:189.
41. Menon DK, Coles JP, Gupta AK, et al. Diffusion limited oxygen delivery following head injury. Crit Care Med 2004;32:1384.
42. Nortje J, Coles JP, Timofeev I, et al. Effect of hyperoxia on regional oxygenation and metabolism after severe traumatic brain injury: preliminary findings. Crit Care Med 2008;36:273.
43. Pickard JD, Hutchinson PJ, Coles JP, et al. Imaging of cerebral blood flow and metabolism in brain injury in the ICU. Acta Neurochir Suppl 2005;95:459.
44. Ricker JH, Muller RA, Zafonte RD, et al. Verbal recall and recognition following traumatic brain injury: a [0-15]-water positron emission tomography study. J Clin Exp Neuropsychol 2001;23:196.
45. Steiner LA, Coles JP, Johnston AJ, et al. Responses of posttraumatic pericontusional cerebral blood flow and blood volume to an increase in cerebral perfusion pressure. J Cereb Blood Flow Metab 2003;23:1371.

46. Vespa P, Bergsneider M, Hattori N, et al. Metabolic crisis without brain ischemia is common after traumatic brain injury: a combined microdialysis and positron emission tomography study. J Cereb Blood Flow Metab 2005;25:763.
47. Ikeda Y, Long DM. The molecular basis of brain injury and brain edema: the role of oxygen free radicals. Neurosurgery 1990;27:1.
48. Schmidley JW. Free radicals in central nervous system ischemia. Stroke 1990;21:1086.
49. Bergsneider M, Hovda DA, McArthur DL, et al. Metabolic recovery following human traumatic brain injury based on FDG-PET: time course and relationship to neurological disability. J Head Trauma Rehabil 2001;16:135.
50. Langfitt TW, Obrist WD, Alavi A, et al. Computerized tomography, magnetic resonance imaging, and positron emission tomography in the study of brain trauma. Preliminary observations. J Neurosurg 1986;64:760.
51. Allen-Auerbach M, Weber WA. Measuring response with FDG-PET: methodological aspects. Oncologist 2009;14:369.
52. Bastiaannet E, Hoekstra OS, Oyen WJ, et al. Level of fluorodeoxyglucose uptake predicts risk for recurrence in melanoma patients presenting with lymph node metastases. Ann Surg Oncol 2006;13:919.
53. Bastiaannet E, Oyen WJ, Meijer S, et al. Impact of [18F]fluorodeoxyglucose positron emission tomography on surgical management of melanoma patients. Br J Surg 2006;93:243.
54. Benz MR, Allen-Auerbach MS, Eilber FC, et al. Combined assessment of metabolic and volumetric changes for assessment of tumor response in patients with soft-tissue sarcomas. J Nucl Med 2008;49:1579.
55. Duch J, Fuster D, Munoz M, et al. 18F-FDG PET/CT for early prediction of response to neoadjuvant chemotherapy in breast cancer. Eur J Nucl Med Mol Imaging 2009;36:1551.
56. Furth C, Steffen IG, Amthauer H, et al. Early and late therapy response assessment with [18F]fluorodeoxyglucose positron emission tomography in pediatric Hodgkin's lymphoma: analysis of a prospective multicenter trial. J Clin Oncol 2009;27:4385.
57. Jacene HA, Filice R, Kasecamp W, et al. 18F-FDG PET/CT for monitoring the response of lymphoma to radioimmunotherapy. J Nucl Med 2009;50:8.
58. Roedl JB, Colen RR, Holalkere NS, et al. Adenocarcinomas of the esophagus: response to chemoradiotherapy is associated with decrease of metabolic tumor volume as measured on PET-CT. Comparison to histopathologic and clinical response evaluation. Radiother Oncol 2008;89:278.
59. Roedl JB, Halpern EF, Colen RR, et al. Metabolic tumor width parameters as determined on PET/CT predict disease-free survival and treatment response in squamous cell carcinoma of the esophagus. Mol Imaging Biol 2009;11:54.
60. Schwarz JK, Grigsby PW, Dehdashti F, et al. The role of 18F-FDG PET in assessing therapy response in cancer of the cervix and ovaries. J Nucl Med 2009;50(Suppl 1):64S.
61. Votrubova J, Belohlavek O, Jaruskova M, et al. The role of FDG-PET/CT in the detection of recurrent colorectal cancer. Eur J Nucl Med Mol Imaging 2006;33:779.
62. Yao M, Graham MM, Smith RB, et al. Value of FDG PET in assessment of treatment response and surveillance in head-and-neck cancer patients after intensity modulated radiation treatment: a preliminary report. Int J Radiat Oncol Biol Phys 2004;60:1410.
63. Yao M, Smith RB, Graham MM, et al. The role of FDG PET in management of neck metastasis from head-and-neck cancer after definitive radiation treatment. Int J Radiat Oncol Biol Phys 2005;63:991.
64. Zhang HQ, Yu JM, Meng X, et al. Prognostic value of serial [(18)F]fluorodeoxyglucose PET-CT uptake in stage III patients with non-small cell lung cancer treated by concurrent chemoradiotherapy. Eur J Radiol 2009. [Epub ahead of print].
65. Ratain MJ, Eckhardt SG. Phase II studies of modern drugs directed against new targets: if you are fazed, too, then resist RECIST. J Clin Oncol 2004;22:4442.
66. Wahl RL, Jacene H, Kasamon Y, et al. From RECIST to PERCIST: Evolving Considerations for PET response criteria in solid tumors. J Nucl Med 2009;50(Suppl 1):122S.
67. Dubroff JG, Ficicioglu C, Segal S, et al. FDG-PET findings in patients with galactosaemia. J Inherit Metab Dis 2008;31:533.
68. Kang KW, Lee DS, Cho JH, et al. Quantification of F-18 FDG PET images in temporal lobe epilepsy patients using probabilistic brain atlas. Neuroimage 2001;14:1.
69. Signorini M, Paulesu E, Friston K, et al. Rapid assessment of regional cerebral metabolic abnormalities in single subjects with quantitative and nonquantitative [18F]FDG PET: A clinical validation of statistical parametric mapping. Neuroimage 1999;9:63.
70. Kraus MF, Smith GS, Butters M, et al. Effects of the dopaminergic agent and NMDA receptor antagonist amantadine on cognitive function, cerebral glucose metabolism and D2 receptor availability in chronic traumatic brain injury: a study using positron emission tomography (PET). Brain Inj 2005;19:471.
71. Takasawa M, Beech JS, Fryer TD, et al. Imaging of brain hypoxia in permanent and temporary middle cerebral artery occlusion in the rat using 18F-fluoromisonidazole and positron emission tomography: a pilot study. J Cereb Blood Flow Metab 2007;27:679.

72. Saita K, Chen M, Spratt NJ, et al. Imaging the ischemic penumbra with 18F-fluoromisonidazole in a rat model of ischemic stroke. Stroke 2004;35:975.
73. Spratt NJ, Ackerman U, Tochon-Danguy HJ, et al. Characterization of fluoromisonidazole binding in stroke. Stroke 2006;37:1862.
74. Spratt NJ, Donnan GA, Howells DW. Characterisation of the timing of binding of the hypoxia tracer FMISO after stroke. Brain Res 2009;1288:135.
75. Choi SR, Golding G, Zhuang Z, et al. Preclinical properties of 18F-AV-45: a PET agent for Abeta plaques in the brain. J Nucl Med 2009;50:1887.
76. Jagust WJ, Landau SM, Shaw LM, et al. Relationships between biomarkers in aging and dementia. Neurology 2009;73:1193.
77. Kemppainen NM, Aalto S, Wilson IA, et al. PET amyloid ligand [11C]PIB uptake is increased in mild cognitive impairment. Neurology 2007;68:1603.
78. Scheinin NM, Aalto S, Koikkalainen J, et al. Follow-up of [11C]PIB uptake and brain volume in patients with Alzheimer disease and controls. Neurology 2009;73:1186.
79. Brody DL, Magnoni S, Schwetye KE, et al. Amyloid-beta dynamics correlate with neurological status in the injured human brain. Science 2008;321:1221.
80. De Beaumont L, Theoret H, Mongeon D, et al. Brain function decline in healthy retired athletes who sustained their last sports concussion in early adulthood. Brain 2009;132:695.
81. McKee AC, Cantu RC, Nowinski CJ, et al. Chronic traumatic encephalopathy in athletes: progressive tauopathy after repetitive head injury. J Neuropathol Exp Neurol 2009;68:709.
82. Chen MK, Guilarte TR. Translocator protein 18 kDa (TSPO): molecular sensor of brain injury and repair. Pharmacol Ther 2008;118:1.
83. Jansen HM, van der Naalt J, van Zomeren AH, et al. Cobalt-55 positron emission tomography in traumatic brain injury: a pilot study. J Neurol Neurosurg Psychiatr 1996;60:221.
84. Szelies B, Sobesky J, Pawlik G, et al. Impaired benzodiazepine receptor binding in peri-lesional cortex of patients with symptomatic epilepsies studied by [(11)C]-flumazenil PET. Eur J Neurol 2002;9:137.
85. Venneti S, Wagner AK, Wang G, et al. The high affinity peripheral benzodiazepine receptor ligand DAA1106 binds specifically to microglia in a rat model of traumatic brain injury: implications for PET imaging. Exp Neurol 2007;207:118.

PET in Epilepsy and Other Seizure Disorders

Abass Alavi, MD*, Andrew B. Newberg, MD

KEYWORDS

- Positron emission tomography • Neurophysiology
- Epilepsy • Seizure disorders

Epilepsy affects 0.5% to 1.0% of the population and can cause focal, partial, generalized, and absence seizures in addition to several more unusual types. Seizure disorders often begin in childhood and are treated with a variety of anticonvulsant medications or surgery for those refractory to medical therapy. Functional imaging, with PET and single-photon emission computed tomography (SPECT), has been useful in the diagnosis, management, and follow-up of patients with seizure disorders. The ability of functional neuroimaging to provide important information about seizures is based on the physiologic alterations in the brain caused by epileptic conditions. These physiologic changes occur during seizures and between seizures. Because generalized seizures affect a large part of the brain, it may be more difficult to isolate the originating focus from other areas that are secondarily affected on functional imaging studies. However, for partial seizures, as well as other seizure types that originate from a specific focus, functional neuroimaging with PET can be useful for localizing the primary site. PET imaging also helps in the understanding of the pathophysiology of seizure disorders. This article reviews the literature regarding the current uses and indications for PET in the study and management of patients with seizure disorders.

PET imaging in particular has been used in the management of patients with seizure disorders in the past 2 decades. In general, during an epileptic seizure, cerebral metabolism and cerebral blood flow (CBF) are markedly increased. During the interictal period, cerebral metabolism and CBF are decreased.[1] In patients with generalized seizures, interictal [^{18}F]fluorodeoxyglucose (FDG)-PET studies do not show focal areas of hypometabolism.[2] However, the focus of partial seizures (with or without secondary generalized seizures) can frequently be identified using FDG-PET because the seizure focus will have increased metabolic activity during the seizure that is less than normal levels in the interictal state.[3–8] It has been shown that single hypometabolic regions can be identified in 55% to 80% of patients with focal surface electroencephalography (EEG) abnormalities.[4,9,10] These areas of decreased metabolism often appear more extensive than anatomic abnormalities observed on magnetic resonance (MR) imaging.[1,11] Interictal PET is also a useful technique in patients with an unlocalized surface ictal EEG seizure focus. Therefore, PET can be used to reduce the number of invasive EEG studies in patients with seizure disorders.[12,13]

INTERICTAL PET IMAGING

Interictal PET scanning has been used in a variety of seizure disorders and for several different purposes. The most commonly studied disorders include temporal lobe epilepsy (TLE) and frontal lobe seizures. Interictal PET scans [14] in patients with complex partial seizures showed that only the duration of the seizure disorder correlated with the degree of interhemispheric asymmetry in glucose metabolism and blood flow compared with other clinical parameters such as age at seizure onset, frequency of complex partial

Division of Nuclear Medicine, Department of Radiology, Hospital of the University of Pennsylvania, 110 Donner Building, 3400 Spruce Street, Philadelphia, PA 19104, USA
* Corresponding author.
E-mail address: abass.alavi@uphs.upenn.edu

PET Clin 5 (2010) 209–221
doi:10.1016/j.cpet.2010.03.001

seizures, history of secondary generalization, history of febrile seizures, and MR imaging evidence for mesial temporal sclerosis. However, the degree of asymmetry was significantly greater for glucose uptake than for blood flow, suggesting that there is an uncoupling of metabolism and blood flow that is a progressive process. This uncoupling may result from the differential response of glucose metabolism and blood flow to chronic seizure activity. Another study of a single patient with bifrontal seizures found improvement in metabolic abnormalities after medical control of the seizures.[15] However, in contrast to the 2 reports described earlier, a further study did not find any association between complex partial seizure frequency or lifetime number of secondarily caused generalized seizures and hippocampal volume or metabolism.[16] These investigators concluded that the progression of metabolic or pathologic abnormalities may not be altered by adequate seizure control. Thus, simply the presence of an epileptic focus might be associated with progressive neuronal injury even if the patient may be well controlled medically.

Several confounding clinical issues that may affect global or regional cerebral metabolism, such as the types of seizures, time since the last seizure, concomitant depression or neuropsychiatric disorders (**Fig. 1**), and medication use (**Fig. 2**), require consideration in the evaluation of PET scans. Because it is not clear which factors play a role in the metabolic landscape of patients with complex partial seizures, Savic and colleagues[17] investigated whether the metabolic pattern of interictal PET may be related to the EEG and clinical features of the seizure that preceded the scan. For this study, patients were classified into 4 groups focal limbic (characterized by aurae or staring spells), widespread limbic (including automatisms), complex partial seizures with posturing, and secondarily generalized seizures. This study showed that hypometabolism

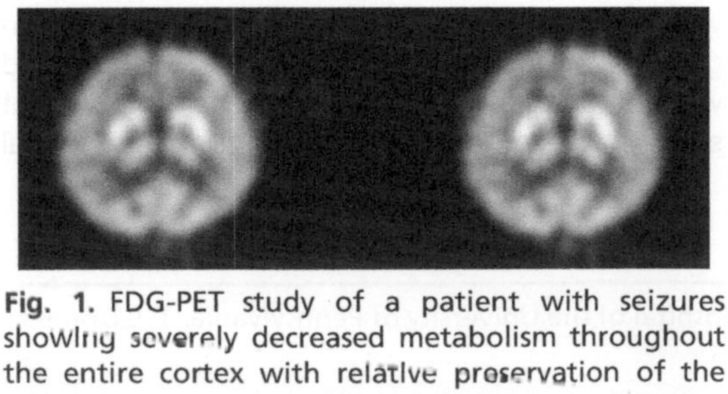

Fig. 1. FDG-PET study of a patient with seizures showing severely decreased metabolism throughout the entire cortex with relative preservation of the subcortical structures. This study does not localize a seizure focus and is more consistent with depression or selected psychopharmacologic agents.

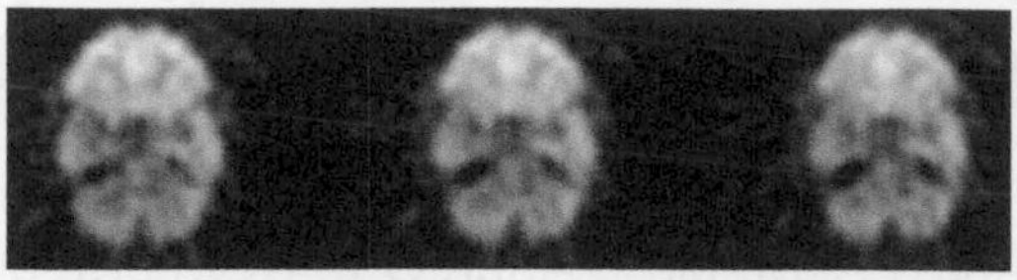

Fig. 2. Interictal FDG-PET study from a patient with seizures. A specific seizure focus could not be identified, but there is bilaterally decreased metabolism in the cerebellum. This finding is common in patients on antiseizure medications such as Dilantin.

was limited to the epileptogenic zone if the preceding seizure was focal limbic, whereas patients with widespread limbic seizures had hypometabolism that included 1 or several additional areas of the limbic cortex. Patients with posturing were found to have hypometabolism in the extralimbic frontal lobe. Patients with secondarily generalized seizures were found to have significant cerebellar and parietal hypometabolism. The results of this study suggested that the mechanisms involved in the generation of a seizure that precedes a PET scan influences the interictal hypometabolic pattern and that it is important to consider the type of nonhabitual seizure that precedes a PET scan when interpreting images.

A study by Barrington and colleagues[18] used simultaneous scalp EEG during FDG administration to determine the exact ictal or interictal state of the patient with intractable seizures. This study found that seizures occur infrequently during FDG administration and that concurrent scalp EEG may not be necessary unless there is a significant problem with interpretation of the PET scan. Another study compared interictal regional slow activity (IRSA) as measured by scalp EEG with FDG-PET imaging and showed that the presence of such EEG activity had a high correlation with temporal lobe hypometabolism.[19] IRSA was not specifically related to mesial temporal sclerosis or any other pathology. The investigators suggested that the findings from this study indicate that the hypometabolism observed on PET may delineate a region of reduced neuronal inhibition that can receive interictal and ictal propagation.

Most patients with epilepsy respond to medical therapy. However, some patients are found to be refractory to such treatments. One FDG-PET study in adolescents showed that detection of hypometabolism in the area of the seizure focus is associated with a poorer response to drug treatment compared with those without such findings.[20] In patients refractory to medical interventions, in the pediatric and adult populations, one of the most effective treatments for partial epilepsy is surgical removal of the involved area. Using high-resolution PET images, accurate localization of seizure foci can be achieved to aid in selecting the appropriate candidates for surgical intervention.[3–5,8,21] Studies have also found that, after surgical excision of the seizure focus, there is usually significant improvement in the function of the rest of the brain.[22] This is true in seizures associated with cortical dysplasia, which typically present at a younger age and have greater seizure frequency compared with most seizures from other causes. Cortical dysplasia is the most frequent seizure cause in patients younger than 18 years, but is the third most common cause behind hippocampal sclerosis and tumors in adult epilepsy surgery patients.[23] In a recent review of multiple studies in the literature, FDG-PET imaging was found to be positive in 75% to 90% of patients with cortical dysplasia.[24]

In terms of specific brain structures, the temporal lobe is the most common focus of partial epilepsy (**Figs. 3** and **4**). Initial studies showed that the sensitivity of PET in detecting TLE seizure focus is more than 70%.[25–35] A more recent study has shown that FDG-PET findings led clinicians to change the surgical decision they had made based on MR imaging and video-EEG monitoring findings in 71%.[36] In 17% of all referred patients, the decision regarding surgical candidacy was based on FDG-PET findings. FDG-PET provided the most additional benefit when previous MR imaging results were normal or did not show unilateral temporal abnormalities, or when ictal EEG results were not consistent with MR imaging findings. However, a recent meta-analysis suggested that ipsilateral hypometabolism may be an indicator for good postoperative outcome in the presurgical evaluation of TLE patients, but the diagnostic added value was questionable and unclear.[37] Another issue with regard to diagnosis is that false lateralization can occur with PET imaging, reflected as hypometabolism of the temporal lobe contralateral to the site of seizure focus as determined by EEG or MR imaging.[38] However, this is not a common phenomenon, as reflected in the

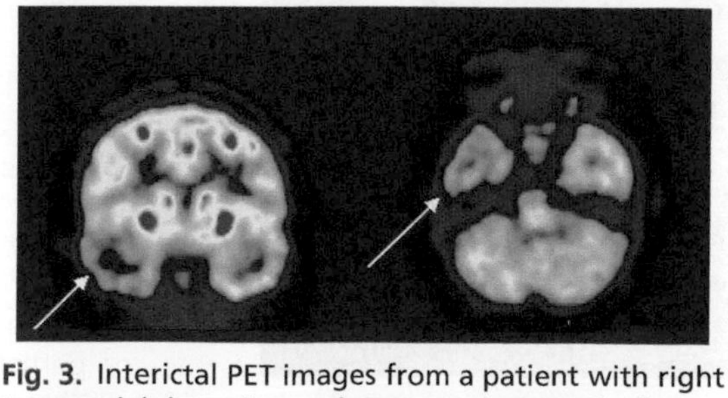

Fig. 3. Interictal PET images from a patient with right temporal lobe seizure shown as decreased glucose metabolism in the right temporal lobe (*arrow*).

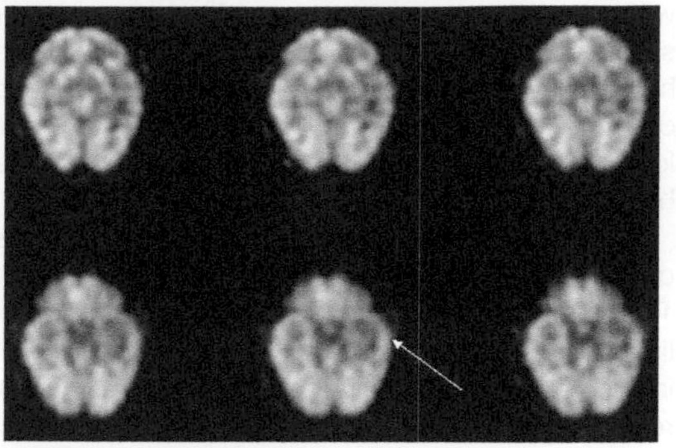

Fig. 4. Interictal PET images from a patient with left temporal lobe seizure shown as decreased glucose metabolism in the left temporal lobe (*arrow*).

sensitivity and specificity of PET for detecting seizure foci. PET imaging is also useful in detecting metabolic abnormalities in pediatric patients, suggesting that focal functional deficits appear early in patients, especially those with medically refractory TLE.[39] Thus, PET imaging may help in the early identification of these patients.

Newer methods for analyzing PET images have also been explored, such as statistical parametric mapping (SPM), in which each pixel represents a z-score value determined by using the mean and standard deviation of count distribution in each individual patient. A study using SPM compared hemispheric asymmetry on FDG-PET images in patients who had mesial TLE with controls.[40] When the SPM program was used to detect temporal interhemispheric asymmetry, hypometabolism was identified on the side chosen for resection in most cases (sensitivity, 71%; specificity, 100%) and was predictive of favorable postsurgical outcome in 90% of the patients. After a correction for multiple comparisons, SPM also identified temporal lobe hypermetabolic areas as well as extratemporal cortical and subcortical hypometabolic areas on the side of resection and on the contralateral side. An analysis of interictal FDG-PET scans in 17 patients with surgically treated TLE showed that the mean z-scores were significantly more negative in anterolateral and mesial regions on the operated side than on the nonoperated side in those patients who were seizure free, but not in those with ongoing seizures postoperatively.[41] SPM correctly lateralized 16 of 17 patients, but only the anterolateral region was significant in predicting surgical outcome. Another study also reported that SPM analysis may help identify bitemporal lobe hypometabolism better than visual assessment alone.[42] A more recent study of 46 patients showed that voxel-based analysis of FDG scans revealed hypometabolism in the epileptogenic cortex that was correlated with the duration of seizures.[43] Several other studies also confirmed the ability of FDG-PET to help predict postsurgical seizure outcome based on the degree of hypometabolism in the temporal lobes[44] and the extent of resection of the hypometabolic area.[45]

PET studies have also shown changes in areas distant from the seizure focus in patients with TLE. One FDG-PET study showed hypometabolism of the seizure focus in the temporal pole, but increased metabolism in the ipsilateral mesiobasal region.[46] Contralateral to the seizure focus, metabolism was increased in the lateral temporal cortex and mesiobasal regions. A study of patients with bilateral TLE found that approximately 10% of the PET scans from such patients had bilateral temporal lobe hypometabolism.[47] Patients with bilateral temporal lobe hypometabolism had a higher percentage of generalized seizures, were more likely to have bilateral, diffuse, or extratemporal seizure onsets, and had bilateral or diffuse MR imaging findings, compared with patients with unilateral temporal lobe hypometabolism. Medical treatment was also less successful in patients with bilateral temporal lobe hypometabolism, and these patients also had worse social and cognitive functioning. Patients with bilateral temporal lobe hypometabolism had a worse prognosis for seizure remission after surgery. A more recent study showed that patients with bilateral temporal lobe hypometabolism had more frequent nonlateralized ictal EEG pattern, anterior temporal white-matter changes, and less frequent aura and unilateral dystonic posturing.[48] However, this study showed no substantial difference in postoperative outcomes between patients with bilateral or unilateral temporal lobe involvement on PET.

Another important aspect of seizure studies is how to distinguish those patients who will do well postoperatively from those who will be less likely to benefit from temporal lobectomy. In this regard, PET studies have yielded controversial results. One PET study did not find any correlation between the severity of abnormal temporal lobe blood flow and the frequency of postoperative seizures.[49] However, this study had a limited number of patients and may not have been able to detect statistical differences. Other studies have shown that in those patients with hypometabolism only in the affected temporal lobe, there is a higher likelihood of a successful outcome.[41,50,51] It has also been shown that patients with a greater degree of temporal lobe hypometabolism (ie, a more distinct asymmetry) tend to have a better outcome than those with a lesser degree of asymmetry.[51–53] It may be that those patients without significant hypometabolism of the affected temporal lobe (ie, minimal asymmetry between the temporal lobes) might have extratemporal or bitemporal seizure foci. These patients may therefore be less amenable to surgical resection. This possibility is corroborated by other studies that have shown that patients with hypometabolism in the contralateral hemisphere to the epileptic focus on EEG may be more likely to have postoperative seizures,[54,55] and those patients with extratemporal hypometabolism tend to have a higher likelihood of postoperative seizures (**Fig. 5**).[50,56]

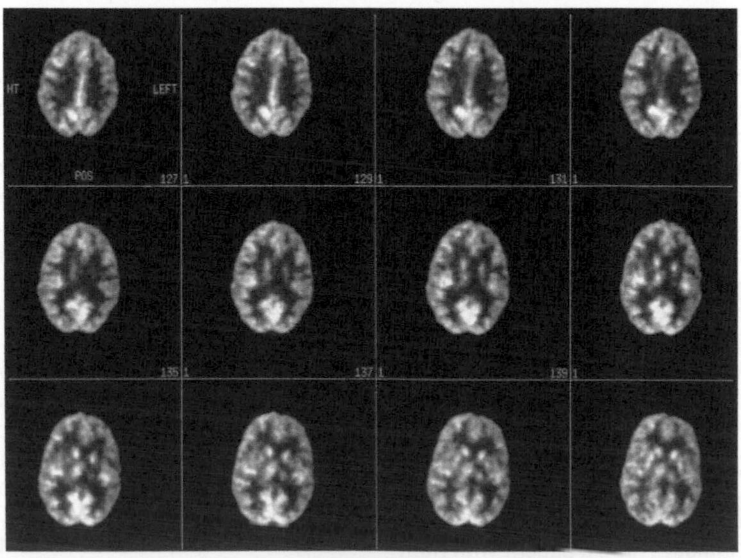

Fig. 5. Interictal FDG-PET study of a patient showing hypometabolism in the entire left hemisphere including the thalamus and basal ganglia. A specific seizure focus could not be identified.

Several studies have indicated that those patients with mesial temporal hypometabolism on PET imaging have a higher probability of being free of seizures postoperatively than those patients with hypometabolism in other parts of the temporal lobe.[53] Other studies have suggested that lateral temporal lobe hypometabolism is a good predictor of a seizure-free postoperative outcome.[12,52] Despite the findings regarding the association of temporal lobe hypometabolism with postoperative seizure outcome, several studies have not shown such a relationship.[57] Other studies using discriminant and multivariate analysis have confirmed that temporal lobe hypometabolism was a good predictor of postoperative seizure outcome.[58] Furthermore, a study comparing MR imaging and PET found that patients with white-matter changes on MR imaging in the temporal lobes had greater reductions in glucose metabolism in the same regions.[59] These patients also had better postsurgical outcomes, suggesting that MR imaging and PET findings can be used in a complementary manner.

The thalamus may be an important structure to evaluate in patients with TLE regarding postoperative seizure outcome. The findings from one study suggest that metabolic dysfunction of the thalamus ipsilateral to the seizure focus becomes more severe with long-standing temporal or frontal lobe epilepsy (FLE), and with secondary generalization of seizures.[60] One article showed that of 64 patients who were seizure free postoperatively, all had either no thalamic metabolic asymmetry or had asymmetry in the same direction as that of the temporal lobe removed (ie, the thalamus ipsilateral to the temporal lobe hypometabolism appeared to have reduced metabolism).[61] No patients who were seizure free had thalamic asymmetry in the reverse direction to that of the temporal lobe removed (ie, the thalamus contralateral to the temporal lobe hypometabolism appeared to have reduced metabolism). In contrast, 5/16 patients (31%) with postoperative seizures of any degree had thalamic asymmetry in the reverse direction to that of the temporal lobe removed. All 5 patients with this reverse thalamic asymmetry were found to have some degree of postoperative seizure. This study has been corroborated by a more recent report of 36 patients in which 90% of patients with ipsilateral thalamic hypometabolism obtained a good seizure outcome, whereas only 40% of those with contralateral thalamic hypometabolism had a good outcome.[62] Contralateral thalamic hypometabolism as a predictor of poor postoperative seizure outcome may be taken to reflect a widespread pattern of seizure activity. However, despite persistent seizures in patients with reverse thalamic asymmetry, there was still some degree of seizure activity improvement. Therefore, although the finding of reverse thalamic asymmetry may provide important prognostic information, surgery can still be an effective intervention in such patients.

PET imaging has also been used after surgical interventions to determine the postoperative metabolic landscape. A study of 8 patients undergoing temporal lobectomy had follow-up PET scans at least 6 months after surgery.[63] Half of the patients showed improved glucose metabolism in the formerly hypometabolic areas that were remote to the surgical site and ipsilateral to the epileptogenic foci. Patients who showed bilateral temporal hypometabolism preoperatively had contralateral temporal hypometabolism after surgery. Several areas, particularly the frontal lobes, showed increased glucose metabolism after surgery. The investigators concluded that hypometabolism in remote areas ipsilateral to the seizure focus may show reversibility after surgery, and thus may be caused by inhibition via the intercortical pathways. This conclusion has been confirmed more recently in a study of 15 patients with seizure disorders,[64] in which postoperative glucose metabolism increased in extratemporal areas ipsilateral to the affected side, particularly in the frontal cortices, bilateral inferior parietal lobules, and in the remaining temporal lobe regions remote from the resected mesial temporal region. By contrast, postoperative glucose metabolism decreased only in the mesial temporal area adjacent to the resected region. Contralateral temporal hypometabolic areas that persist after surgery may be caused by a different mechanism, and neither specifically indicates the presence of a seizure foci nor affects the seizure outcome. PET imaging in a patient after entorhinoamygdalohippocampectomy performed with γ-knife surgery showed relative improvement in metabolism in the lateral temporal lobe with persistently decreased metabolism in the mesial temporal lobe.[65]

The other major site of the seizure focus in partial epilepsy is the frontal lobe (**Fig. 6**). Because

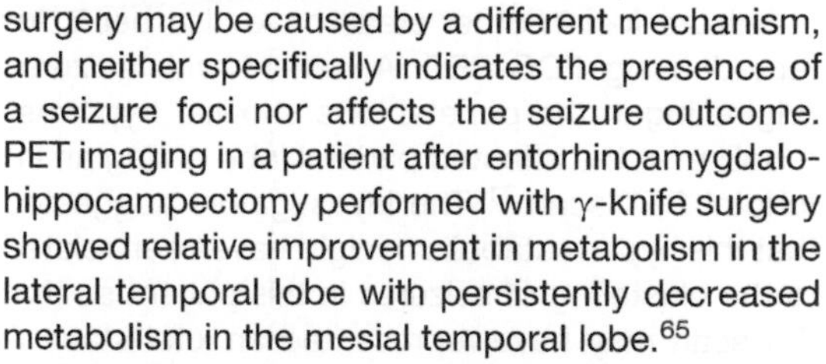

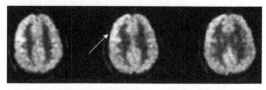

Fig. 6. Ictal FDG-PET study of a patient showing hypermetabolism in the right frontal lobe (*arrow*) compared with the rest of the cortical areas. This study indicates a seizure focus in the right frontal lobe.

many of these seizures begin in the medial or inferior aspects of the frontal lobe, scalp EEG readings frequently do not provide adequate localization of foci.[66,67] Franck and colleagues[33] used interictal FDG-PET to study 13 patients with presumed FLE and found PET to be the best modality for localizing seizure foci in this location. The investigators suggested that PET might help in determining the site of surgical excision or suggest a contraindication to surgical intervention in patients with multiple or bilateral foci. A study of 180 surgical specimens from patients with FLE found a high correlation between hypometabolic regions on interictal PET images and structural, histopathologic changes in the surgical specimens.[68] This study was corroborated by an earlier study in which FDG-PET images revealed decreased frontal lobe metabolism in 64% of patients with frontal lobe seizures as determined by electroclinical ictal localization.[69] A study of pediatric patients showed a similar sensitivity of FDG-PET in detecting frontal lobe seizure foci.[70] However, PET scans showed hypometabolism restricted to the frontal lobes in approximately 62%. The remaining patients showed hypometabolism that extended beyond the epileptogenic region indicated by ictal EEG. Although extrafrontal hypometabolism has an uncertain cause in these patients, this finding may be the result of additional epileptogenic areas, effects of diaschisis, seizure propagation sites, or secondary epileptogenic foci. Regardless, the findings from the studies on FLE suggest that FDG-PET scanning is a useful technique for investigating patients with seizures of probable frontal lobe origins.

Seizure foci in other areas have also been detected using FDG-PET. A patient with seizures originating in the parietal lobe showed hypermetabolism in the affected parietal lobe during an interictal PET scan.[71] The investigators suggested that this hypermetabolism might have been related to the clustering of seizures in this patient so that the scan may have represented an ictal state. A more recent evaluation of parietal lobe seizures found that the sensitivity for detecting the seizure focus was comparable for MR imaging, PET, and SPECT, although MR imaging was the highest at approximately 64%, whereas PET had a sensitivity of only 50%.[72] The results indicate that parietal lobe seizures are much more difficult to localize than temporal or frontal lobe seizures.

Interictal FDG-PET imaging has generally been shown to be useful in detecting seizure foci and helping to predict prognosis. It is a technique that has also been shown to be a cost-effective measure in the presurgical evaluation of patients with seizure disorders.[73] It is probably most useful in the setting of equivocal findings on MR imaging or video-EEG.

ICTAL PET IMAGING

Performing ictal PET studies is logistically more difficult than interictal studies because of the short half-life of positron-emitting isotopes such as fluorine 18.[74] The short half-life makes it difficult to have a standing dose available for injection at the initiation of seizure activity on EEG. However, several ictal PET studies have been reported to have been successful in the determination of seizure foci in patients with partial seizures. In these studies, the seizure focus appears as a hypermetabolic area. In earlier studies, Chugani and colleagues[75] devised a classification system to describe the metabolic patterns observed in children with partial complex seizures. Specifically, 3 major metabolic patterns were observed and were based on the degree and type of subcortical involvement. The type I pattern was defined as asymmetric glucose metabolism of the striatum and thalamus. Patients with this pattern often showed unilateral cortical and crossed cerebellar hypermetabolism. The type II pattern included symmetric hypermetabolism in the striatum and thalamus that was associated with hypermetabolism of the hippocampus or insular cortex. The type II pattern also included diffuse cortical hypometabolism and the absence of any cerebellar abnormalities. The type III pattern showed hypermetabolism that was restricted to the cerebral cortex with normal metabolism in the striatum and thalamus. Despite defining these 3 patterns of FDG-PET findings, this study could not correlate the PET findings with EEG or clinical features of the seizure disorders in these patients.

Another ictal PET study using $H_2{}^{15}O$ showed that complex partial seizures are associated with bilaterally increased CBF in several cortical areas, particularly the temporal and frontal lobes.[76] In addition, these patients also had increased blood flow to the subcortical areas that are activated during ictus.

SURGICAL PLANNING WITH PET

Several studies have used PET imaging for the specific purpose of planning surgical interventions. Duncan and colleagues[77] used $H_2{}^{15}O$ PET in conjunction with anatomic images from MR imaging to determine the brain regions involved with motor activity, visual perception, articulation, and receptive language tasks in pediatric patients before temporal, and even extratemporal, surgery. At follow-up, the patients who underwent temporal lobectomy and extratemporal resection for a neoplastic or nonneoplastic seizure focus were seizure free with minimal postoperative morbidity. The investigators noted that no child sustained a postoperative speech or language deficit. When patients had prenatal cortical injury, PET showed reorganization of language areas to new, adjacent areas or even to the contralateral hemisphere. One study used ictal PET overlayed onto the corresponding anatomic MR imaging to successfully determine the seizure focus and to help with neurosurgical planning.[78] Cognitive activation paradigms using PET imaging has been suggested as an alternative approach to the evaluation of functional and epileptogenic regions for presurgical evaluation in patients with epilepsy.[79] More work is needed to determine the most clinically efficacious paradigms for different seizure types. The investigators suggest that the strength of activation PET studies lies in the ability to study shifts in cognitive circuitry that accompany a fixed neuropathologic entity for groups of similar subjects and individuals. These techniques may enhance our understanding of the fundamentals of brain plasticity and may be used in the future to predict precise surgical risks.

By combining PET and MR imaging data, these studies show an enhancement in surgical safety, definition of optimal surgical approach, delineation of the seizure focus, and facilitation of maximum resection and optimization of the timing of surgery. Thus, noninvasive presurgical brain mapping with PET can reduce the risk and improve neurologic outcome in patients with seizure disorders undergoing surgical resection.

RECEPTOR PET IMAGING

PET imaging of various neurotransmitter systems has been used in the study of patients with seizure disorders. Initial studies of benzodiazepine receptor activity in TLE showed decreased benzodiazepine receptor activity in the medial temporal lobe.[80] This reduction in benzodiazepine receptor activity may correlate with the frequency of seizures.[81] A more recent study compared the results obtained from FDG and [^{11}C]flumazenil.[82] FDG-PET images showed a large area of hypometabolism in the epileptogenic temporal lobe (as determined by other diagnostic studies including scalp EEG and MR imaging). FDG-PET and [^{11}C]flumazenil PET reliably revealed the epileptogenic temporal lobe and neither agent proved superior. This study did not find any correlation between the degree of hypoactivity in [^{18}F]FDG or [^{11}C]flumazenil PET and the grading of mesial temporal sclerosis according to the Wyler criteria observed with MR imaging. Furthermore, this study compared the PET results with those obtained with interictal [^{123}I]iomazenil SPECT and found that the latter was highly inaccurate in localizing the affected temporal lobe. It has been suggested that, in the pediatric population, [^{11}C]flumazenil PET may have a useful clinical role in patients with partial epilepsy who have equivocal findings on FDG-PET, in patients with bilateral FDG findings but unifocal seizure activity on EEG, and in patients after surgical resection who continue to have seizures.[83] This latter group often have large areas of hypometabolism on FDG-PET in the area of the resection that may also include remaining epileptogenic foci.

Another study compared changes in benzodiazepine receptors in the thalami of patients with TLE.[84] The dorsal medial nuclei showed significantly lower glucose metabolism and [^{11}C]flumazenil binding on the side of the epileptic focus. The lateral thalami showed bilateral hypermetabolism and increased [^{11}C]flumazenil binding. A significant correlation was found between the [^{11}C]flumazenil binding in the dorsal medial nuclei and that in the amygdala. These PET abnormalities were associated with a significant volume loss in the ipsilateral thalamus as determined by anatomic MR imaging. Decreased benzodiazepine receptor binding in the dorsal medial nucleus may be to the result of neuronal loss, as suggested by volume loss on MR imaging, but this decrease may also indicate impaired γ-aminobutyric acid (GABA)ergic transmission in the dorsal medial nucleus, which has strong reciprocal connections with other parts of the limbic system. The increased glucose metabolism and [^{11}C]flumazenil binding in the lateral thalamus was hypothesized to represent an upregulation of GABA-mediated inhibitory neural circuits. FLE is associated with significantly reduced benzodiazepine receptor density in the anterior cerebellum contralateral to the seizure focus.[85]

A study using [^{11}C]flumazenil for 6 patients with frontal lobe seizures[86] reported that the seizure focus was correctly identified by [^{11}C]flumazenil PET as an area of decreased benzodiazepine receptor density in all patients studied. The area with reduced benzodizepine receptor density was better delineated than the corresponding hypometabolic region observed with FDG-PET images. Several other studies of benzodiazepine receptors showed that the areas of abnormal receptor binding were more extensive than anatomic abnormalities observed on MR imaging, or even than the hypometabolic areas observed on interictal FDG-PET.[87,88]

Several studies have shown the involvement of the opioid neurotransmitter systems in seizure physiology. Several PET studies using the δ-receptor-selective antagonist [^{11}C]methylnaltrindole and the μ-opiate receptor tracer, [^{11}C]carfentanil in patients with TLE have shown increased receptor activity in the affected temporal lobe.[89–91] Compared with interictal FDG-PET, the binding of opiate receptors was increased and FDG uptake decreased in the temporal cortex ipsilateral to the seizure focus.[91] Furthermore, decreases in FDG uptake were more widespread than the increases in opioid receptors. There were also different regional binding patterns for the δ and μ receptors. Increases in μ-receptor binding were localized to the middle aspect of the inferior temporal lobe and binding of δ receptors increased in the middle and superior temporal lobe. There are differences in the regional binding of the μ- and δ-opiate receptors, which suggests that they may play different roles in seizure physiology. A recent study of [^{11}C]diprenorphine (nonspecific opioid binding) by Hammers and colleagues[92] showed increased postictal [^{11}C]diprenorphine binding. The investigators suggested that synaptic opioid levels increase at the time of seizures, which is followed by a gradual recovery of available surface receptors with an overshoot compared with basal levels. This overshoot was detected by PET about 8 hours after the seizure. These results suggested an important role for the opioid system in the postictal increase in seizure threshold.

Recent studies imaging the serotonergic system also indicate a potential use in detecting seizure foci. For example, a recent study in patients with TLE using [^{18}F]2′-methoxyphenyl-(*N*-2′-pyridinyl)-*p*-fluoro-benzamidoethyipiperazine (MPPF) PET data, visual evaluation blinded to clinical information yielded a sensitivity of 90% (38 of 42 patients) for detecting the seizure focus, even in those patients without hippocampal sclerosis. This study suggested that imaging the 5-hydroxytryptamine 1A (5-HT_{1A}) receptor with [^{18}F]MPPF PET might be valuable in the preoperative evaluation of patients with TLE.[93] Another study suggested that imaging the 5-HT_{1A} receptor may be a better modality than FDG-PET in patients with TLE negative on MR imaging.[94]

OTHER SEIZURE DISORDERS

There are several other seizure disorders that have been investigated using PET imaging. Absence seizures are a common form of epilepsy associated with brief spells of loss of consciousness. These seizures are associated with 3-Hz generalized spike-wave activity on EEG. The site of the absence seizure origin has been difficult to detect and localize. A $H_2{}^{15}O$ PET CBF study was performed on 8 patients with idiopathic generalized epilepsy in whom typical absence seizures were induced by voluntary hyperventilation.[95] This study showed that there was a global increase in blood flow during the typical absence seizures. There was also a focal increase in mean thalamic blood flow. However, although it indicated an important role of the thalamus in the pathogenesis of absence seizures, this study was unable to show that the thalamus was the origin of the seizure activity. An ictal FDG-PET study of patients in absence status showed decreased metabolic rates throughout cortical and subcortical structures compared with interictal scans.[2] A comparison with single absence attacks suggested that there is a pathophysiologic difference between the 2 states. A recent case study reported localizing absence seizures in 1 patient to the right frontal lobe using ictal PET.[96] No evidence was found for a change in [^{11}C]flumazenil binding with absence seizures. This result, together with those of a study showing no abnormality of [^{11}C]flumazenil binding interictally in patients with childhood and juvenile absence epilepsy, does not support a primary role for the benzodiazepine binding site of the GABA-A receptor in the pathogenesis of absence seizures.[97]

Another unusual epileptic disorder consists of focal inhibitory motor seizures that result in ictal paralysis. A study of this type of seizure disorder showed that these patients had a centroparietal epileptogenic focus on SPECT that was also suggested by other neuroimaging studies.[98] In particular, MR imaging showed centroparietal structural lesions in most of the patients. In 1 patient with a normal MR imaging scan, there was right centroparietal hypometabolism on PET imaging. Given these findings, the investigators suggested that it is important to distinguish such seizures from transient ischemic attacks and migraine, which may not have the same imaging findings.

Infantile spasms may occur due to an underlying, identifiable cause (symptomatic group) or may be idiopathic (cryptogenic group). PET studies have found that cryptogenic spasms have focal cortical regions of hypometabolism in the interictal period.[99,100] The focal areas found on PET correspond to areas of EEG abnormalities in these patients. A recent study suggested that there are multifocal areas of hypometabolism in such patients and that the structures involved are associated with specific disease characteristics.[101] For example, frontal hypometabolism correlated with the degree of mental retardation, hypotonia, and ataxia. Temporomesial hypometabolism correlated with the occurrence of obtunded states and parietal changes were associated with the occurrence of myoclonic seizures and spike-wave discharges. Because of the poor prognosis of infants with infantile spasm, surgical removal of the abnormal foci identified by PET has been attempted. The results indicate that 75% of the patients will remain seizure free, whereas others improved markedly after surgery.[102,103]

Lenox-Gastaut syndrome, the triad of 1- to 2.5-Hz spike-wave pattern on EEG, intellectual impairment, and multiple seizure types, has been investigated with PET and 4 patterns have been described.[104,105] The 4 metabolic subtypes are unilateral focal, unilateral diffuse and bilateral diffuse hypometabolism, and normal metabolism.[106,107] Because this disorder is often refractory to anticonvulsant therapy, surgical intervention has been attempted with subsequent control of seizure activity.[108] Therefore, PET imaging may provide useful information regarding the type of surgical intervention necessary in these patients.[105] Another study of Lennox-Gastaut syndrome found that PET scans were normal in all children with typical de novo Lennox-Gastaut syndrome, but showed cortical metabolic abnormalities in 3/4 with atypical de novo Lennox-Gastaut syndrome, 5/6 with Lennox-Gastaut syndrome following infantile spasms, 6/8 with severe myoclonic epilepsy in infancy, and 4/6 with an unclassified epileptic encephalopathy.[109] The findings from this study suggest that some children with epileptic encephalopathies previously believed to have primary generalized or multifocal seizures may have a unifocal origin for their seizures. If a focal origin is observed, then surgical intervention may be useful as a treatment modality in these cases. Patients with Sturge-Weber syndrome, characterized by facial capillary nevus (port-wine stain) and ipsilateral leptomeningeal angiomatosis, often develop epileptic seizures due to the intracranial, extracerebral vascular malformation. Like infantile spasms and Lenox-Gastaut syndrome, Sturge-Weber syndrome is usually refractory to medications and requires surgical intervention. In conjunction with computed tomography (CT) and MR imaging, PET has been useful in helping to determine the surgical technique (usually a hemispherectomy) necessary in these patients.[103] PET imaging usually shows widespread unilateral hypometabolism ipsilateral to the facial nevus.[105] As with other seizure disorders, hypermetabolism is noted ipsilateral to the facial nevus during the ictal period.

SUMMARY

PET imaging has been widely used in the evaluation and management of patients with seizure disorders. The ability of PET to measure cerebral function makes it ideal for studying the neurophysiologic correlates of seizure activity during ictal and interictal states. PET imaging is also useful for evaluating patients before surgical interventions to determine the best surgical method and maximize outcomes. Thus, PET will continue to play a major role not only in the clinical arena but also in further investigations of the pathogenesis and management of various seizure disorders.

REFERENCES

1. Duncan JS. Imaging and epilepsy. Brain 1997; 120(Pt 2):339–77.
2. Theodore WH, Brooks R, Margolin R, et al. Positron emission tomography in generalized seizures. Neurology 1985;35(5):684–90.
3. Abou-Khalil BW, Siegel GJ, Sackellares JC, et al. Positron emission tomography studies of cerebral glucose metabolism in chronic partial epilepsy. Ann Neurol 1987;22:480–6.
4. Engel J Jr, Brown WJ, Kuhl DE, et al. Pathologic findings underlying focal temporal lobe hypometabolism in partial epilepsy. Ann Neurol 1982;12: 518–28.
5. Engel J Jr, Kuhl DE, Phelps ME, et al. Comparative localization of the epileptic foci in partial epilepsy by PET and EEG. Ann Neurol 1982;12:529–37.
6. Engel J Jr, Kuhl DE, Phelps ME, et al. Local cerebral metabolism during partial seizures. Neurology 1983;33:400–13.
7. Theodore WH, Brooks R, Sato S, et al. The role of positron emission tomography in the evaluation of seizure disorders. Ann Neurol 1984;15(Suppl): S176–9.
8. Theodore WH, Newmark ME, Sato S, et al. 18F fluorodeoxyglucose positron emission tomography in refractory complex partial seizures. Ann Neurol 1983;13:537.
9. Engel J Jr. PET scanning in partial epilepsy. Can J Neurol Sci 1991;18(Suppl):588–92.
10. Duncan R. Epilepsy, cerebral blood flow, and cerebral metabolic rate. Cerebrovasc Brain Metab Rev 1992;4:105–21.
11. Theodore WH, Holmes MD, Dorwart RH, et al. Complex partial seizures: cerebral structure and cerebral function. Epilepsia 1986;27(5):576–82.
12. Theodore WH, Sato S, Kufta CV, et al. FDG-positron emission tomography and invasive EEG: seizure focus detection and surgical outcome. Epilepsia 1997;38(1):81–6.
13. Debets RM, van Veelen CW, Maquet P, et al. Quantitative analysis of 18/FDG-PET in the presurgical evaluation of patients suffering from refractory partial epilepsy. Comparison with CT, MRI, and

combined subdural and depth EEG. Acta Neurochir Suppl (Wien) 1990;50:88–94.
14. Breier JI, Mullani NA, Thomas AB, et al. Effects of duration of epilepsy on the uncoupling of metabolism and blood flow in complex partial seizures. Neurology 1997;48(4):1047–53.
15. Matheja P, Weckesser M, Debus O, et al. Drug-induced changes in cerebral glucose consumption in bifrontal epilepsy. Epilepsia 2000;41(5): 588–93.
16. Spanaki MV, Kopylev L, Liow K, et al. Relationship of seizure frequency to hippocampus volume and metabolism in temporal lobe epilepsy. Epilepsia 2000;41(9):1227–9.
17. Savic I, Altshuler L, Baxter L, et al. Pattern of interictal hypometabolism in PET scans with fludeoxyglucose F 18 reflects prior seizure types in patients with mesial temporal lobe seizures. Arch Neurol 1997;54(2):129–36.
18. Barrington SF, Koutroumanidis M, Agathonikou A, et al. Clinical value of "ictal" FDG-positron emission tomography and the routine use of simultaneous scalp EEG studies in patients with intractable partial epilepsies. Epilepsia 1998 Jul;39(7):753–66.
19. Koutroumanidis M, Binnie CD, Elwes RD, et al. Interictal regional slow activity in temporal lobe epilepsy correlates with lateral temporal hypometabolism as imaged with 18FDG PET: neurophysiological and metabolic implications. J Neurol Neurosurg Psychiatr 1998;65(2):170–6.
20. Gaillard WD, White S, Malow B, et al. FDG-PET in children and adolescents with partial seizures: role in epilepsy surgery evaluation. Epilepsy Res 1995;20(1):77–84.
21. Utsubo H, Chuang SH, Hwang PA, et al. Neuroimaging for investigation of seizures in children. Pediatr Neurosurg 1992;18:105–16.
22. Verity CM, Strauss EH, Moyes PD, et al. Long-term follow-up after cerebral hemispherectomy. Neurophysiologic, radiologic, and psychological findings. Neurology 1982;32:629–39.
23. Becker AJ, Blumcke I, Urbach H, et al. Molecular neuropathology of epilepsy-associated glioneuronal malformations. J Neuropathol Exp Neurol 2006;65:99–108.
24. Lerner JT, Salamon N, Hauptman JS, et al. Assessment and surgical outcomes for mild type I and severe type II cortical dysplasia: a critical review and the UCLA experience. Epilepsia 2009;50(6): 1310–35.
25. Engel J Jr, Kuhl DE, Phelps ME. Patterns of human local cerebral glucose metabolism during epileptic seizures. Science 1982;218:64–6.
26. Markand ON, Salanova V, Worth R, et al. Comparative study of interictal PET and ictal SPECT in complex partial seizures. Acta Neurol Scand 1997;95:129–36.
27. Boling WW, Lancaster M, Kraszpulski M, et al. Fluorodeoxyglucose-positron emission tomographic imaging for the diagnosis of mesial temporal lobe epilepsy. Neurosurgery 2008;63(6):1130–8.
28. Theodore WH, Dorwart R, Holmes M, et al. Neuroimaging in refractory partial seizures. comparison of PET, CT, and MRI. Neurology 1986;36:750–9.
29. Theodore WH, Fishbein D, Dubinsky R. Patterns of cerebral glucose metabolism in patients with partial seizures. Neurology 1988;38:1201–6.
30. Kuhl DE, Engel J, Phelps ME, et al. Epileptic pattern of local cerebral metabolism and perfusion in human determined by emission computed tomography of ^{18}FDG and $^{13}NH_3$. Ann Neurol 1979;8:348–60.
31. Salanova V, Morris HH 3rd, Rehm P, et al. Comparison of the intracarotid amobarbital procedure and interictal cerebral 18-fluorodeoxyglucose positron emission tomography scans in refractory temporal lobe epilepsy. Epilepsia 1992;33(4):635–8.
32. Bernardi S, Trimble MR, Frackowiak RSJ, et al. An interictal study of partial epilepsy using positron emission tomography and oxygen 15 inhalation method. J Neurol Neurosurg Psychiatr 1983;46: 473–7.
33. Franck G, Maquet P, Sadzot B, et al. Contribution of positron emission tomography to the investigation of epilepsies of frontal lobe origin. Adv Neurol 1992;57:471–85.
34. Salanova V, Markand O, Worth R, et al. FDG-PET and MRI in temporal lobe epilepsy: relationship to febrile seizures, hippocampal sclerosis and outcome. Acta Neurol Scand 1998;97(3): 146–53.
35. Knowlton RC, Laxer KD, Ende G, et al. Presurgical multimodality neuroimaging in electroencephalographic lateralized temporal lobe epilepsy. Ann Neurol 1997;42:829–37.
36. Uijl SG, Leijten FS, Arends JB, et al. The added value of [18F]-fluoro-D-deoxyglucose positron emission tomography in screening for temporal lobe epilepsy surgery. Epilepsia 2007;48(11): 2121–9.
37. Willmann O, Wennberg R, May T, et al. The contribution of 18F-FDG PET in preoperative epilepsy surgery evaluation for patients with temporal lobe epilepsy: a meta-analysis. Seizure 2007;16(6): 509–20.
38. Nagarajan L, Schaul N, Eidelberg D, et al. Contralateral temporal hypometabolism on positron emission tomography in temporal lobe epilepsy. Acta Neurol Scand 1996;93(2–3):81–4.
39. Salanova V, Markand O, Worth R, et al. Presurgical evaluation and surgical outcome of temporal lobe epilepsy. Pediatr Neurol 1999;20(3):179–84.
40. Van Bogaert P, Massager N, Tugendhaft P, et al. Statistical parametric mapping of regional glucose

metabolism in mesial temporal lobe epilepsy. Neuroimage 2000;12(2):129–38.

41. Wong CY, Geller EB, Chen EQ, et al. Outcome of temporal lobe epilepsy surgery predicted by statistical parametric PET imaging. J Nucl Med 1996; 37(7):1094–100.
42. Kim MA, Heo K, Choo MK, et al. Relationship between bilateral temporal hypometabolism and EEG findings for mesial temporal lobe epilepsy: analysis of 18F-FDG PET using SPM. Seizure 2006;15(1):56–63.
43. Akman CI, Ichise M, Olsvasky A, et al. Epilepsy duration impacts on brain glucose metabolism in temporal lobe epilepsy: results of voxel-based mapping. Epilepsy Behav 2010;17(3):373–80.
44. Lin TW, de Aburto MA, Dahlbom M, et al. Predicting seizure-free status for temporal lobe epilepsy patients undergoing surgery: prognostic value of quantifying maximal metabolic asymmetry extending over a specified proportion of the temporal lobe. J Nucl Med 2007;48(5):776–82.
45. Vinton AB, Carne R, Hicks RJ, et al. The extent of resection of FDG-PET hypometabolism relates to outcome of temporal lobectomy. Brain 2007; 130(Pt 2):548–60.
46. Rubin E, Dhawan V, Moeller JR, et al. Cerebral metabolic topography in unilateral temporal lobe epilepsy. Neurology 1995;45(12):2212–23.
47. Blum DE, Ehsan T, Dungan D, et al. Bilateral temporal hypometabolism in epilepsy. Epilepsia 1998;39(6):651–9.
48. Joo EY, Lee EK, Tae WS, et al. Unitemporal vs bitemporal hypometabolism in mesial temporal lobe epilepsy. Arch Neurol 2004;61(7):1074–8.
49. Theodore WH, Gaillard WD, Sato S, et al. Positron emission tomographic measurement of cerebral blood flow and temporal lobectomy. Ann Neurol 1994;36(2):241–4.
50. Manno EM, Sperling MR, Ding X, et al. Predictors of outcome after anterior temporal lobectomy: positron emission tomography. Neurology 1994;44(12): 2331–6.
51. Radtke RA, Hanson MW, Hoffman JM, et al. Temporal lobe hypometabolism on PET: predictor of seizure control after temporal lobectomy. Neurology 1993;43(6):1088–92.
52. Theodore WH, Sato S, Kufta C, et al. Temporal lobectomy for uncontrolled seizures: the role of positron emission tomography. Ann Neurol 1992; 32:789–94.
53. Delbeke D, Lawrence SK, Abou-Khalil BW, et al. Postsurgical outcome of patients with uncontrolled complex partial seizures and temporal lobe hypometabolism on 18FDG-positron emission tomography. Invest Radiol 1996;31:261–6.
54. Benbadis SR, So NK, Antar MA, et al. The value of PET scan (and MRI and Wada test) in patients with bitemporal epileptiform abnormalities. Arch Neurol 1995;52(11):1062–8.
55. Choi JY, Kim SJ, Hong SB, et al. Extratemporal hypometabolism on FDG PET in temporal lobe epilepsy as a predictor of seizure outcome after temporal lobectomy. Eur J Nucl Med Mol Imaging 2003;30(4):581–7.
56. Swartz BE, Tomiyasu U, Delgado-Escueta AV, et al. Neuroimaging in temporal lobe epilepsy: test sensitivity and relationships to pathology and postoperative outcome. Epilepsia 1992;33(4):624–34.
57. Theodore WH, Katz D, Kufta C, et al. Pathology of temporal lobe foci: correlation with CT, MRI and PET. Neurology 1990;40:797–803.
58. Dupont S, Semah F, Clemenceau S, et al. Accurate prediction of postoperative outcome in mesial temporal lobe epilepsy: a study using positron emission tomography with 18fluorodeoxyglucose. Arch Neurol 2000;57(9):1331–6.
59. Choi D, Na DG, Byun HS, et al. White-matter change in mesial temporal sclerosis: correlation of MRI with PET, pathology, and clinical features. Epilepsia 1999;40(11):1634–41.
60. Benedek K, Juhasz C, Muzik O, et al. Metabolic changes of subcortical structures in intractable focal epilepsy. Epilepsia 2004;45(9):1100–5.
61. Newberg AB, Alavi A, Berlin J, et al. Ipsilateral and contralateral thalamic hypometabolism as a predictor of outcome after temporal lobectomy for seizures. J Nucl Med 2000;41(12):1964–8.
62. Sakamoto S, Takami T, Tsuyuguchi N, et al. Prediction of seizure outcome following epilepsy surgery: asymmetry of thalamic glucose metabolism and cerebral neural activity in temporal lobe epilepsy. Seizure 2009;18(1):1–6.
63. Akimura T, Yeh HS, Mantil JC, et al. Cerebral metabolism of the remote area after epilepsy surgery. Neurol Med Chir (Tokyo) 1999;39(1):16–25 [discussion: 25–7].
64. Takaya S, Mikuni N, Mitsueda T, et al. Improved cerebral function in mesial temporal lobe epilepsy after subtemporal amygdalohippocampectomy. Brain 2009;132(Pt 1):185–94.
65. Regis J, Semah F, Bryan RN, et al. Early and delayed MR and PET changes after selective temporomesial radiosurgery in mesial temporal lobe epilepsy. AJNR Am J Neuroradiol 1999;20(2): 213–6.
66. Lee JJ, Lee SK, Lee SY, et al. Frontal lobe epilepsy: clinical characteristics, surgical outcomes and diagnostic modalities. Seizure 2008;17(6):514–23.
67. Quesney LF, Olivier A, Andermann F, et al. Preoperative EEG investigation in patients with frontal lobe epilepsy. trends, results and pathophysiological considerations. J Clin Neurophysiol 1987;4:208–9.
68. Robitaille Y, Rasmussen T, Dubeau F, et al. Histopathology of nonneoplastic lesions in frontal lobe

epilepsy. Review of 180 cases with recent MRI and PET correlations. Adv Neurol 1992;57:499–511.
69. Swartz BE, Halgren E, Delgado-Escueta AV, et al. Neuroimaging in patients with seizures of probable frontal lobe origin. Epilepsia 1989;30(5): 547–58.
70. da Silva EA, Chugani DC, Muzik O, et al. Identification of frontal lobe epileptic foci in children using positron emission tomography. Epilepsia 1997; 38(11):1198–208.
71. Oka A, Kubota M, Sakakihara Y, et al. A case of parietal lobe epilepsy with distinctive clinical and neuroradiological features. Brain Dev 1998;20(3): 179–82.
72. Kim DW, Lee SK, Yun CH, et al. Parietal lobe epilepsy: the semiology, yield of diagnostic workup, and surgical outcome. Epilepsia 2004; 45(6):641–9.
73. O'Brien TJ, Miles K, Ware R, et al. The cost-effective use of 18F-FDG PET in the presurgical evaluation of medically refractory focal epilepsy. J Nucl Med 2008;49(6):931–7.
74. Alavi A, Hirsch LJ. Studies of central nervous system disorders with single photon emission computed tomography and positron emission tomography. Evolution over the past 2 decades. Semin Nucl Med 1991;21:58–81.
75. Chugani HT, Rintahaka PJ, Shewmon DA. Ictal patterns of cerebral glucose utilization in children with epilepsy. Epilepsia 1994;35(4):813–22.
76. Theodore WH, Balish M, Leiderman D, et al. Effect of seizures on cerebral blood flow measured with $^{15}O-H_2O$ and positron emission tomography. Epilepsia 1996;37(8):796–802.
77. Duncan JD, Moss SD, Bandy DJ, et al. Use of positron emission tomography for presurgical localization of eloquent brain areas in children with seizures. Pediatr Neurosurg 1997;26(3):144–56.
78. Meltzer CC, Adelson PD, Brenner RP, et al. Planned ictal FDG PET imaging for localization of extratemporal epileptic foci. Epilepsia 2000;41(2): 193–200.
79. Swartz BE, Mandelkern MA. Positron emission tomography: the contribution of cognitive activation paradigms to the understanding of the epilepsies. Adv Neurol 1999;79:901–15.
80. Savic I, Persson A, Roland P, et al. In-vivo demonstration of reduced benzodiazepine receptor binding in human epileptic foci. Lancet 1988;2: 863–6.
81. Savic I, Svanborg E, Thorell JO. Cortical benzodiazepine receptor changes are related to frequency of partial seizures: a positron emission tomography study. Epilepsia 1996;37(3):236–44.
82. Debets RM, Sadzot B, van Isselt JW, et al. Is 11C-flumazenil PET superior to 18FDG PET and 123I-iomazenil SPECT in presurgical evaluation of temporal lobe epilepsy? J Neurol Neurosurg Psychiatr 1997;62(2):141–50.
83. Chugani HT, Chugani DC. Basic mechanisms of childhood epilepsies: studies with positron emission tomography. Adv Neurol 1999;79:883–91.
84. Juhasz C, Nagy F, Watson C, et al. Glucose and (11C)flumazenil positron emission tomography abnormalities of thalamic nuclei in temporal lobe epilepsy. Neurology 1999;53(9):2037–45.
85. Savic I, Thorell JO. Localized cerebellar reductions in benzodiazepine receptor density in human partial epilepsy. Arch Neurol 1996;53(7): 656–62.
86. Savic I, Thorell JO, Roland P. (11C)flumazenil positron emission tomography visualizes frontal epileptogenic regions. Epilepsia 1995;36(12): 1225–32.
87. Arnold S, Berthele A, Drzezga A, et al. Reduction of benzodiazepine receptor binding is related to the seizure onset zone in extratemporal focal cortical dysplasia. Epilepsia 2000;41(7):818–24.
88. Richardson MP, Koepp MJ, Brooks DJ, et al. Benzodiazepine receptors in focal epilepsy with cortical dysgenesis: an 11C-flumazenil PET study. Ann Neurol 1996;40(2):188–98.
89. Fisher RS, Frost JJ. Epilepsy. J Nucl Med 1991;32: 651–9.
90. Frost JJ, Mayhberg HS, Fisher RS, et al. Mu-opiate receptors measured by positron emission tomography are increased in temporal lobe epilepsy. Ann Neurol 1988;23:231–7.
91. Madar I, Lesser RP, Krauss G, et al. Imaging of delta- and mu-opioid receptors in temporal lobe epilepsy by positron emission tomography. Ann Neurol 1997;41(3):358–67.
92. Hammers A, Asselin MC, Hinz R, et al. Upregulation of opioid receptor binding following spontaneous epileptic seizures. Brain 2007;130(Pt 4): 1009–16.
93. Didelot A, Ryvlin P, Lothe A, et al. PET imaging of brain 5-HT1A receptors in the preoperative evaluation of temporal lobe epilepsy. Brain 2008;131: 2751–64.
94. Liew CJ, Lim YM, Bonwetsch R, et al. 18F-FCWAY and 18F-FDG PET in MRI-negative temporal lobe epilepsy. Epilepsia 2009;50(2):234–9.
95. Prevett MC, Duncan JS, Jones T, et al. Demonstration of thalamic activation during typical absence seizures using $H_2(15)O$ and PET. Neurology 1995; 45(7):1396–402.
96. Millan E, Abou-Khalil B, Delbeke D, et al. Frontal localization of absence seizures demonstrated by ictal positron emission tomography. Epilepsy Behav 2001;2(1):54–60.
97. Prevett MC, Lammertsma AA, Brooks DJ, et al. Benzodiazepine-GABAA receptor binding during absence seizures. Epilepsia 1995;36:592–9.

98. Abou-Khalil B, Fakhoury T, Jennings M, et al. Inhibitory motor seizures: correlation with centroparietal structural and functional abnormalities. Acta Neurol Scand 1995;91(2):103–8.
99. Chugani HT, Shields WD, Shewmon DA, et al. Infantile spasms. I. PET identifies focal cortical dysgenesis in cryptogenic cases for surgical treatment. Ann Neurol 1990;27:406–13.
100. Chugani HT. The use of positron emission tomography in the clinical assessment of epilepsy. Semin Nucl Med 1992;22:247–53.
101. Korinthenberg R, Bauer-Scheid C, Burkart P, et al. 18FDG-PET in epilepsies of infantile onset with pharmacoresistant generalized tonic-clonic seizures. Epilepsy Res 2004;60(1):53–61.
102. Chugani HT, Shewmon DA, Sankar R, et al. Infantile spasms. II. Lenticular nuclei and brain stem activation on positron emission tomography. Ann Neurol 1992;31:212–9.
103. Hoffman HJ, Hendrick EB, Dennis M, et al. Hemispherectomy for Sturge-Weber syndrome. Childs Brain 1979;5:233.
104. Iinuma K, Yanai K, Yanagisawa T, et al. Cerebral glucose metabolism in five patients with Lennox-Gastaut syndrome. Pediatr Neurol 1987;3:12–8.
105. Chugani HT, Mazziotta JC, Phelps ME. Sturge-Weber syndrome. A study of cerebral glucose utilization with positron emission tomography. J Pediatr 1989;114:244–53.
106. Chugani HT, Mazziotta JC, Engel J Jr, et al. Lennox Gastaut syndrome. Metabolic subtypes determined by 18FDG positron emission tomography. Ann Neurol 1987;21:4–13.
107. Theodore WH, Rose D, Patronas N, et al. Cerebral glucose metabolism in the Lennox-Gastaut syndrome. Ann Neurol 1987;21:14–21.
108. Angelini L, Broggi G, Riva D, et al. A case of Lennox-Gastaut syndrome successfully treated by removal of a parietotemporal astrocytoma. Epilepsia 1979;20:665–9.
109. Ferrie CD, Maisey M, Cox T, et al. Focal abnormalities detected by 18FDG PET in epileptic encephalopathies. Arch Dis Child 1996;75:102–7.

Role of PET in the Investigation of Neuropsychiatric Disorders

Andrew B. Newberg, MD*, Abass Alavi, MD

KEYWORDS

- PET • Psychiatric disorders • Depression
- Obsessive-compulsive disorder • Neurotransmitter
- Schizophrenia

PET, along with an array of radiotracers, is used to study many physiologic and pathologic states throughout the body. Its applications in studying the brain, as a research and as a diagnostic clinical tool, have revealed some important findings. Specific psychiatric disorders in which PET studies may influence the management of patients include mood and anxiety disorders, attention deficit disorder, schizophrenia, and obsessive compulsive disorder (OCD).[1]

The only approved radiopharmaceutical for clinical PET imaging is fluorodeoxyglucose (FDG), which measures the cerebral metabolic rate for glucose (**Fig. 1**). There are several other tracers, however, that might be particularly useful in the study of psychiatric disorders. Specifically, tracers that bind to various receptors of neurotransmitter systems, such as serotonin, dopamine, and opiate, may play an important role in the study of psychiatric disorders.[2–9] Other physiologic processes, such as blood flow and amino acid metabolism, might also be relevant. This review of the literature describes the application of PET imaging in the evaluation of a variety of common psychiatric disorders.

DEPRESSION

The most common finding on PET imaging in depressed patients (**Fig. 2**) is a global dysfunction as demonstrated by decreased cerebral blood flow (CBF)[10] and decreased cerebral metabolism.[11] Some studies have indicated that decreased CBF might correlate with the degree of depression. In one group,[12,13] patients with depression had whole-brain decreases in blood flow, with the left anterior cingulate gyrus and the left dorsolateral prefrontal cortex (PFC) particularly affected. Depressed patients who also had cognitive impairment had decreased regional CBF (rCBF) in the left medial frontal gyrus and increased rCBF in the cerebellar vermis compared with depressed patients without cognitive dysfunction. Decreased activity in a localized area in the PFC ventral to the genu of the corpus callosum has been demonstrated in familial bipolar depressives and familial unipolar depressives.[14] Even during non–rapid eye movement sleep, depressed patients have decreased frontal and limbic metabolic activity in association with posterior cortical increases.[15]

An FDG-PET study by Kumar and colleagues[16] showed that patients with late-age onset of depression have decreased metabolism throughout the cortex and even in many subcortical structures. These decreases were of the same or greater magnitude compared with patients with Alzheimer disease. Alzheimer disease patients, however, more likely had the typical temporoparietal hypometabolism pattern on PET images whereas the depression patients tended to have more global hypometabolism.

Division of Nuclear Medicine, Department of Radiology, Hospital of the University of Pennsylvania, 110 Donner Building, 3400 Spruce Street, Philadelphia, PA 19104, USA
* Corresponding author.
E-mail address: Andrew.newberg@uphs.upenn.edu

PET Clin 5 (2010) 223–242
doi:10.1016/j.cpet.2010.03.003
1556-8598/10/$ – see front matter

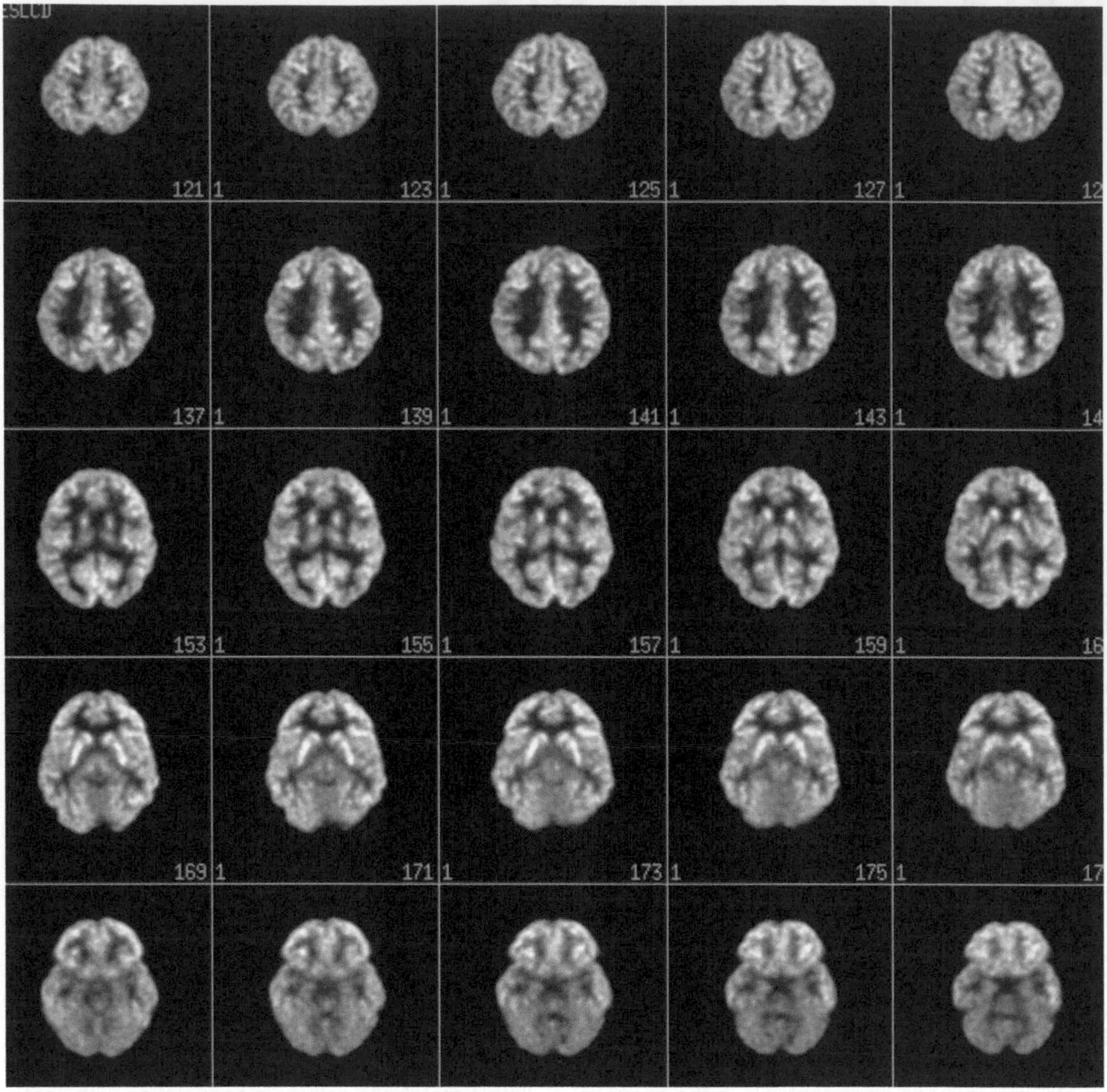

Fig. 1. Normal FDG-PET scan from a healthy individual without any neuropsychiatric disorder. There is uniform distribution of metabolism throughout the cortical and subcortical structures.

Depressed patients with concomitant anxiety symptoms demonstrated specific metabolic changes with increased activity in the right parahippocampal and left anterior cingulate regions and decreased activity in the cerebellum, left fusiform gyrus, left superior temporal, left angular gyrus, and left insula.[17] The investigators concluded that anxiety symptoms are associated with changes in specific brain regions that partially overlap with those in primary anxiety disorders and differ from those associated with depression.

Recent studies have also evaluated treatment-related effects in patients with depression. On pretreatment scans, lower metabolism in the left ventral anterior cingulate gyrus, ventrolateral PFC, orbitofrontal cortex (OFC), and midbrain has been associated with a better treatment response to paroxitine.[18,19] Similarly, other studies have shown that increased metabolism in the ventral anterior cingulate was associated with nonresponse to selective serotonin reuptake inhibitor (SSRI) treatment or cognitive behavioral therapy.[20] There is decreased activity in limbic and striatal areas and increased activity in the dorsal cortical areas (including the prefrontal, parietal, anterior, and posterior cingulated areas) associated with improvements in clinical symptoms.[21] In a study of sleep deprivation, high pretreatment metabolic rates and overall post-treatment decreases in metabolic rates in the medial PFC and anterior cingulated gyrus (particularly on the right) were associated with those

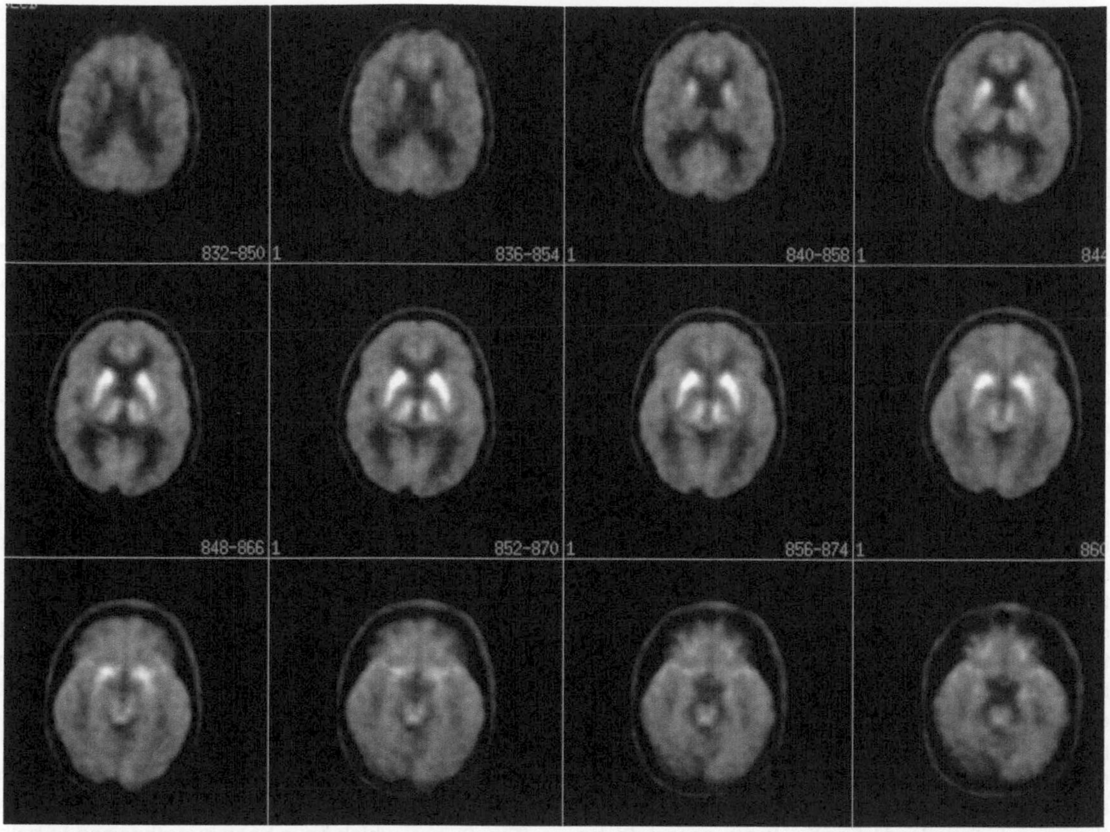

Fig. 2. FDG-PET scan of a patient with major depression showing global cortical decrease in metabolism relative to the subcortical structures.

depression patients who responded well to sleep deprivation therapy.[22,23] In a recent study of nucleus accumbens deep brain stimulation, those patients who responded to the treatment had decreased metabolism in the amygdala and nucleus accumbens.[24]

Another group used PET to study cerebral glucose metabolism in bipolar patients.[25,26] The bipolar patients who were actively depressed had decreased global metabolism. As their depression improved, they had increases in their cerebral metabolism. In contrast, unipolar patients had normal global metabolic rates that did not correlate with clinical symptoms. These investigators also found a decreased caudate to hemispheric metabolic ratio in depressed unipolar patients, and this ratio increased as symptoms of depression improved. Buchsbaum and colleagues[27] found a decreased anteroposterior gradient in bipolar depressed patients but not in unipolar patients. Also, a PET study by Phelps and colleagues[11] reported similar decreases in global metabolism in bipolar patients in the depressive phase, although unipolar patients had global metabolism within normal limits. Furthermore, bipolar patients in the hypomanic phase had normal glucose metabolism. More recent work has demonstrated that unipolar depression is associated with a pattern of prefrontal hypometabolism, whereas a cerebello-posterior cortical hypermetabolism may be observed in bipolar patients. Thus, in depressed patients, PET might be useful in distinguishing unipolar from bipolar patients, a distinction that would have significant implications for a patient's treatment and prognosis.[28]

The serotonin system has been explored particularly in patients with mood disorders because of the effectiveness of SSRIs, which are believed to aid depression by affecting the serotonergic system. The serotonin type 2A receptor does not seem to be affected in late life–onset depression, although there is a decrease in binding to this receptor type in patients with AD.[29] There are typically decreases in serotonergic system, including 1A and 2A receptors in the limbic and neocortical areas.[30–33] A review of serotonin type 2A imaging studies before 2003 of major depressive episodes, however, found a reduction in those depressed patients with recent antidepressant use and no change in those with no recent antidepressant use.[34] The clinical improvement in depressed patients treated with paroxetine was also associated with an increase in the density of serotonin type 2A receptors in the frontal cortex.[35,36] The reduction in serotonin type 1A receptor binding in depressed patients, however, was not changed by SSRI treatment[37] or by electroconvulsive therapy.[38] Also, depressed patients showed a significant reduction in available serotonin type 2A receptors in the brain after desipramine treatment.[39] Serotonin transporter binding measured with ^{11}C-DASB was reduced in the brain stem, thalamus, caudate, putamen, anterior cingulate cortex, and frontal cortex in patients with major depression.[40]

Other receptor types have been studied in patients with mood disorders. Fluorodopa uptake in the left caudate was significantly lower in depressed patients with psychomotor retardation than in patients with high impulsivity and in comparison subjects.[41] A recent study suggests that there is decreased dopamine D2 receptor binding in depression patients after successful electroconvulsive therapy.[42] Some bipolar patients also have psychotic symptoms and had elevations in dopamine D2 receptor density likely associated with the psychotic symptoms and not the mood disorder.[43] Finally, there seems to be decreased γ-aminobutyric acid (GABA)–A binding in the parahippocampus and superior temporal lobe in patients with depression, and the temporal lobe decrease correlated with hypothalamus-pituitary axis hyperactivity.[44]

ANXIETY AND STRESS

PET has been used to attempt to gain a better understanding of the neurophysiologic mechanisms underlying stress and anxiety. In general, the hippocampus, the amygdala, and the PFC as part of the limbic system are believed to play important roles in the regulation of the hypothalamic-pituitary-adrenal axis. Rieman and colleagues[45–47] studied patients with panic disorders using H_2O PET; these patients had increased rCBF in the right parahippocampal gyrus in lactate-vulnerable patients in a resting, nonpanic state, compared with controls (patients in whom intravenous infusion of sodium lactate can induce a panic attack). During a lactate-induced panic attack, the patients had increased rCBF bilaterally in the temporal poles, the claustrum, and the lateral putamen.

In patients with generalized anxiety disorder, there are lower metabolic rates in basal ganglia and white matter and increased metabolism in the left inferior occipital lobe, right posterior temporal lobe, and the right precentral frontal gyrus.[48] In one study, benzodiazepine therapy resulted in decreases in metabolic rates for cortical areas, limbic system, and basal ganglia. A related study showed decreases in metabolism in the visual cortex and increases in the basal ganglia and thalamus.[27] An FDG-PET study found that the PFC is activated in response to psychosocial stress, and distinct prefrontal metabolic glucose patterns are linked to endocrine stress measures, such as cortisol levels.[49]

Patients with simple phobias might also be expected to have changes in cerebral metabolism or blood flow. Mountz and colleagues,[50] however, did not find any changes in these patients in the resting state or when exposed to a phobic stimuli compared with controls. This finding conflicts with the reports of anxiety response in normal patients (discussed previously). Elucidation of the mechanisms underlying anxiety is needed.

Several studies have used PET imaging to evaluate the effects of practices and interventions that might attenuate stress and anxiety. Brain imaging studies suggest that willful acts and tasks that require sustained attention are initiated via activity in the PFC, particularly in the right hemisphere.[51] There is evidence to suggest that during meditation practices, there are frontal lobe increases (**Fig. 3**),[52,53] which have been hypothesized to help modulate activity in the anterior cingulate and limbic structures, possibly resulting in lowering perceived levels of stress, anxiety, and depression.[54]

In terms of neurotransmitter systems, recent PET studies have demonstrated reduced serotonin type 1A receptor binding in patients with panic disorder and social anxiety disorder but not in posttraumatic stress disorder (PTSD).[55] A PET study using ^{11}C-raclopride to measure the dopaminergic tone during Yoga Nidra meditation demonstrated a significant increase in dopamine levels during the meditation practice.[56] The authors hypothesized that this increase may be associated with the gating of cortical-subcortical interactions that leads to an overall decrease in readiness for action associated with this particular type of meditation. Stressors also are shown related to a release of dopamine using PET imaging.[57] Future studies will be necessary to elaborate on the role of dopamine in stress and anxiety.

POSTTRAUMATIC STRESS DISORDER

A few studies have explored cerebral changes associated with PTSD. A case report of a subject exposed to war-related sounds before and after treatment with an SSRI showed that before treatment, trauma reminders resulted in decreased

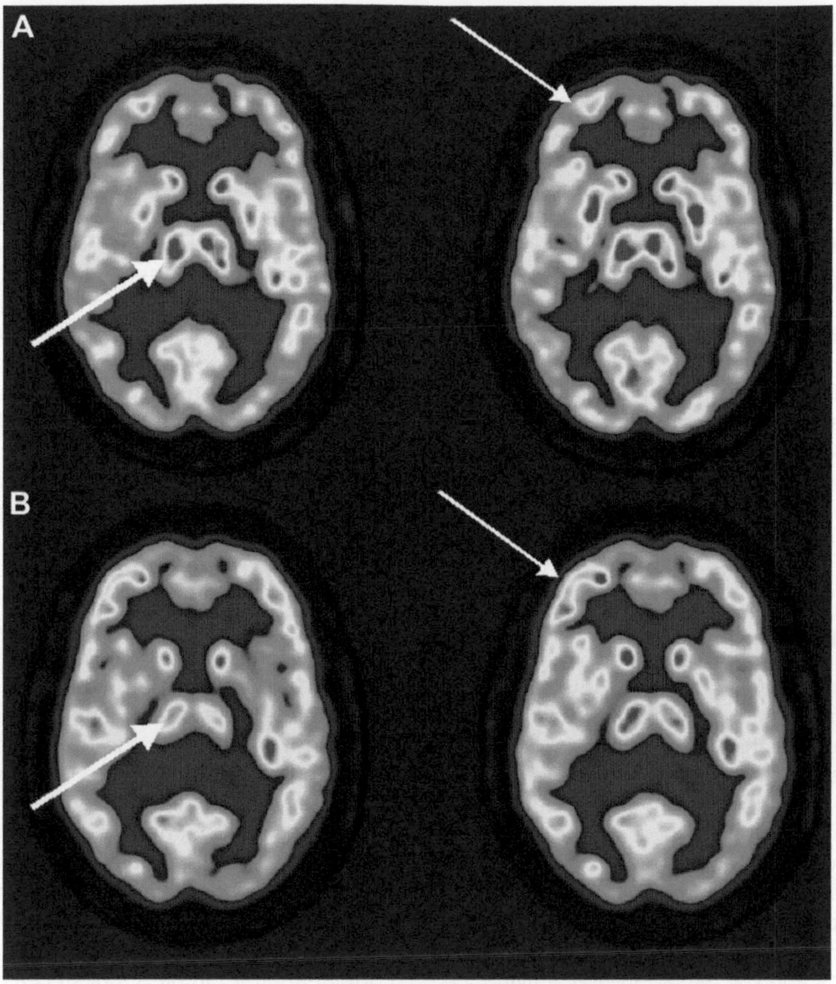

Fig. 3. FDG-PET scans of a subject at rest (*A*) and while performing a meditation task (*B*). During meditation, there is increased metabolism in the frontal lobes (*thin arrow*) and decreased metabolism in the thalami (*thick arrow*). These structures are involved in stress pathways and the observed effects in these scans are hypothesized to be associated reduced levels of stress and anxiety.

rCBF in the insula, prefrontal, and inferior frontal cortices.[58] There was also increased activity in the cerebellum, precuneus, and supplementary motor cortex. These findings normalized after SSRI administration, suggesting that the anxiolytic effect of such medications for PTSD could be mediated by prefrontal and paralimbic cortices, areas typically involved in memory, emotion, attention, and motor control. An FDG-PET study of 15 patients showed that PTSD was associated with diminished activity in the cingulate gyri, precuneus, insula, hippocampus PFC, occipital lobe, and verbal areas.[59] This same study showed increased activity in the fusiform gyrus, superior temporal lobe, and cerebellum in PTSD patients. The amygdala and the thalamus showed normal metabolic activity in this cohort. The investigators suggest that the metabolic pattern was comparable to that in patients with personality disorders of the borderline type.

A different study explored rCBF changes associated with the recollection and imagery of traumatic events in trauma-exposed individuals with and without PTSD.[60] This study showed that the traumatic condition was associated with increases in OFC and anterior temporal poles compared with the neutral condition and that these increases were greater in the PTSD group. rCBF decreases in both anterior frontal regions and the left inferior frontal regions were greater in the PTSD group. A follow-up study by the same group showed that the PTSD group had CBF decreases in the medial frontal gyrus when patients recalled traumatic in comparison with neutral stimulus.[61] CBF changes in medial frontal gyrus were inversely correlated with CBF changes in the amygdala. Symptom severity was positively correlated to CBF in the right amygdala and negatively correlated to CBF in medial frontal gyrus.

Another study explored the association with cocaine and alcohol abuse with PTSD.[62] Such patients had significantly higher rCBF in the right amygdala and the left parahippocampal gyrus than control patients during an auditory continuous performance task. The investigators concluded that the amygdala's attention and fear function suggests that increased amygdala rCBF may be related to clinical features of PTSD. Cocaine use may be associated with increased amygdala rCBF in these PTSD patients. Therefore, the amygdala and frontal cortex attention systems may be reciprocally related and their relative contributions associated with processing of neutral stimuli that are perturbed in patients with cocaine and alcohol abuse in association with PTSD.

SCHIZOPHRENIA

PET has been widely used in the study of the functional abnormalities in schizophrenia.[63–65] It has been suggested that schizophrenia is most commonly associated on PET scans (**Fig. 4**) with frontal lobe dysfunction,[66–69] although other studies did not report such a finding.[70–73] One study showed that the degree of frontal hypometabolism correlated with negative symptoms as opposed to positive symptoms,[74] although other studies have found an association between positive symptoms and decreased frontal activity.[75] A refinement of the proposed hypothesis for the underlying cause of dysfunction in schizophrenia ascribes the hypofrontal pattern to those schizophrenic patients with a predominance of negative symptoms.[76,77] These patients tend to be older and have a long history of neuroleptic therapy. Alternatively, younger patients with predominantly positive symptoms usually have not demonstrated the hypofrontal pattern to the same extent.[78,79] It may also be that the frontal lobe activity changes during the course of the disorder and is more prominent in the acute setting[80] or that frontal lobe changes may vary with specific symptoms in individual patients.[81] There are other areas that may also be affected in schizophrenia, including hypometabolism in the anterior cingulate cortex, striatum, and thalamus.[82–85] Liddle and colleagues[78,79] proposed 3 syndromes of symptoms in schizophrenics with corresponding PET patterns of rCBF: (1) patients with psychomotor poverty syndrome and diminished word-generating ability have decreased perfusion of the dorsolateral PFC; (2) patients with the disorganization syndrome have impaired inhibition of inappropriate responses and have increased rCBF of the right anterior cingulate gyrus; and (3) patients with the reality distortion syndrome have increased perfusion in the medial temporal lobe at a locus that is activated in normal subjects during the internal monitoring of eye movements.

More recent work has tried to establish specific networks of structures related to the clinical manifestations of schizophrenia. For example, there is a correlation between the anterior thalamus and the frontal cortex, a key element in the thalamo-cortical-striatal circuit suggested as abnormal in some models of schizophrenia.[86,87] The findings from this study also showed that schizophrenics

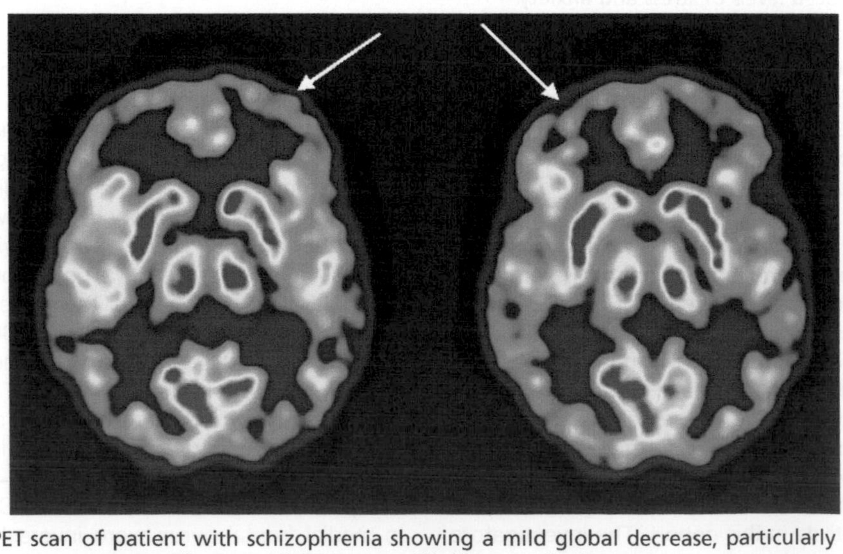

Fig. 4. FDG-PET scan of patient with schizophrenia showing a mild global decrease, particularly in the frontal regions (*arrows*), consistent with some of the reported findings in the literature.

have lower correlations between the frontal lobe activity and that in other structures consistent with frontal cortical dysfunction.

Several PET studies have been performed to determine whether or not left hemispheric dysfunction can be detected in schizophrenics. In some studies, patients with schizophrenia at rest had increased perfusion and metabolism in the left hemispheric cerebral cortex relative to the right.[88–90] Also, the severity of the symptoms of schizophrenia correlated with the degree of hyperactivation of the left hemisphere and not with the degree of hypofrontality. This concurs with a study by Sheppard and colleagues,[91] which found increased blood flow to the left hemisphere using ^{15}O-H_2O PET. Also, Early and colleagues[92] found increased CBF in the left globus pallidus in patients with schizophrenia. Cleghorn and colleagues,[65] however, did not find any significant difference in laterality between schizophrenics and controls. A more recent study showed that patients lack asymmetry in caudate dopamine transporter binding, which conforms with the concept of disrupted brain lateralization in schizophrenia.[93]

Cerebral activation studies have improved the understanding of the cognitive and affective deficits associated with schizophrenia. FDG-PET studies, in which a subject underwent specific frontal lobe activation tests of sustained attention by continuous performance tasks, found decreased activation of the frontal lobes in schizophrenic patients compared with controls.[94,95] DeLisi and colleagues[96] found that schizophrenic patients had higher left temporal lobe metabolic rates compared with controls when there was sensory stimulation of the right arm. Another study[97] compared PET and electroencephalogram findings in schizophrenic and control subjects performing various simple and complex motor tasks. Although no changes were observed in the schizophrenic or control groups during simple motor tasks, the schizophrenic group had decreased activation in the supplementary motor and the contralateral sensorimotor cortices during complex motor tasks compared with controls. During a continuous performance task, schizophrenics showed negative correlations of task performance with anterior cingulate activity, suggesting that overactivity of that region, which is involved in mental effort and whose metabolic rate is typically lower in schizophrenic patients, may also result in the impairment of task performance in these patients.[98] Patients with schizophrenia also fail to activate the anterior cingulate gyrus during selective attention performance.[99] Schizophrenia patients with negative symptoms had a lesser activation in the left hemisphere during word generation with compensatory changes in the right hemisphere.[100] Schizophrenia is also associated with attenuated right thalamic and right prefrontal activation during the recognition of novel visual stimuli and with increased left prefrontal cortical activation during impaired episodic recognition of previously seen visual stimuli.[101] Similarly, patients with schizophrenia fail to activate cortical-cerebellar-thalamic-cortical circuitry during recall of well-learned and novel word lists.[102] Frontal cortex function during memory retrieval is more impaired in schizophenic patients.[103,104] Volkow and colleagues[105] found that with eye-tracking tasks, schizophrenic patients had lower correlations between anterior and posterior cortical areas and between the thalamus and neocortical areas compared with controls. These results suggest a marked derangement in the pattern of interactions between various brain regions in schizophrenics. The results of most of these activation studies suggest abnormal thalamic and PFC function in schizophrenia,[106] although another study showed a cingulate gyrus–parietal lobe dysfunction underlying impairment of working memory processes during a random number generation task in schizophrenia.[107] There has also been evidence of hippocampal dysfunction during episodic memory retrieval in schizophrenia.[108] Schizophrenic patients have also failed to show graded, memory task–related decreases in activity in the left superior temporal and inferior parietal gyrus, which is typically seen in control subjects.[109,110]

In addition to the metabolic and blood flow studies, PET imaging of the dopamine system in schizophrenic patients has been an important advance.[111,112] This is particularly useful because the dopaminergic system has been implicated in the pathophysiology of this disorder as well as the site of action for neuroleptic drugs, the primary therapeutic modality considered effective in these patients. Early studies reported no differences in dopamine receptor density or affinity in the basal striatum between schizophrenics and controls.[113–115] Other studies, however, reported an increased density of dopamine receptors in neuroleptic naive and previously treated but drug-free schizophrenic patients.[116,117] The same group[118] found increases in dopamine activity in patients with manic depressive psychosis suggesting that increased dopamine activity might be a feature of psychotic illness in general and may not be specific to schizophrenia. A recent study using ^{18}F-fallypride showed that in schizophrenic subjects there is increased dopamine D2 receptor levels in the substantia nigra and there was a significant correlation of symptoms of disorganized thinking and nonparanoid delusions with the right temporal cortex binding.[119] In a review article by Howes and colleagues,[120] 6 of 8 studies using ^{18}F-fluorodopa found elevated striatal dopamine uptake in patients with schizophrenia. A recent study also suggests that there is elevated striatal dopamine uptake in patients with prodromal symptoms of schizophrenia as well as in those with frank schizophrenia.[121] These findings suggest that striatal dopamine overactivity predates the onset of schizophrenia. Another study demonstrated that depressive symptoms in neuroleptic-naive, first-admission schizophrenia patients have low presynaptic dopamine function.[122] There has been no evidence of a change in serotonin receptors in patients with schizophrenia,[123,124] although some investigators have reported a decrease in the frontal lobes in neuroleptic-naive patients.[125]

PET studies have also evaluated the effects of therapeutic interventions in patients with schizophrenia. Early studies reported a general increase in glucose metabolism, particularly in the left temporal lobe, after neuroleptic treatment, but there was no change in the anteroposterior gradient.[126,127] Schizophrenic patients who responded to haloperidol treatment typically had a "normalizing" effect on metabolic activity in the striatum, with the metabolic rate when they were receiving haloperidol higher than that when they were receiving placebo.[128] Nonresponders were more likely to show a worsening of hypofrontality and an absence of change in the striatum during the treatment condition. Another study corroborated this finding, in that a haloperidol challenge caused widespread decreases in absolute metabolism in nonresponsive patients but not the responsive patients.[129] Studies have shown that that there is a high dopamine D2 receptor occupancy, particularly in the basal ganglia, in early treatment with neuroleptics, and that this occupancy was dose dependent and associated not only with the therapeutic effect but also with side effects, such as hyperprolactinemia and extrapyramidal signs.[130–132] Upregulation of dopamine D2 receptors has also been associated with a regional increase of blood flow and metabolism in the basal ganglia.[133] Furthermore, the D2 receptor occupancy has been shown to decrease as the drug levels decreased on withdrawal of treatment. Patients who are resistant to neuroleptic therapy have similar D2 receptor blockade compared with patients who respond clinically to therapy.[134,135] In addition to D2 receptor blockade with antipsychotic drugs, Sedvall and colleagues[136] found that there is also blockade of the D1 receptors (D1 receptor activity was measured with ^{11}C–SCH 23390). This is particularly true with the drug clozapine, which shows almost the same amount of D1 as D2 receptor occupancy.[137] The data suggest that traditional and novel antipsychotics with high affinity for dopamine D2 receptors are associated with a substantial increase in D2 receptor binding. The current data in humans corroborate the animal data that implicate D2 receptor-mediated mechanisms in motor hyperactivity.

The atypical antipsychotic, quetiapine, results in a transiently high D2 occupancy, which decreases to low levels by the end of the dosing interval, which may account for its lower incidence of extrapyramidal side effects.[138] Quetiapine and clozapine have a lower incidence of extrapyramidal side effects in part because of their lower striatal D2 binding, whereas their antipsychotic effect may be mediated by preferential binding in the temporal cortex.[139] Another study using ^{11}C-raclopride, however, found that with resperidone and olanzapine, striatal D2 occupancy predicted response in terms of positive psychotic symptoms but not for negative symptoms.[140] PET has also been used to evaluate other new drugs, such as amoxapine and olanzapine, which have a profile similar to that of other atypical antipsychotics with a higher occupancy of serotonin receptors compared with D2 receptors.[141,142] PET imaging has demonstrated gender differences related to the effects with antipsychotic medications with women having a reduction in cingulated gyrus metabolism compared with men with clozapine and fluphenazine.[143] In men, fluphenazine was associated with a greater elevation in basal ganglia metabolic rates than was clozapine whereas women demonstrated nearly equal increases in fluphenazine and clozapine.

OBSESSIVE-COMPULSIVE DISORDER

Several studies have used FDG-PET to investigate patients with OCD. Early results (**Fig. 5**) have generally shown that OCD patients have increased cerebral metabolism in the orbital region of the frontal cortex and the caudate nuclei compared with controls.[144–147] There has not been a consistent observation, however, of increased activity in the caudate. One study also found increased metabolism in the cingulate gyrus of OCD patients compared with controls.[148] PET has been used to explore the effects of different types of therapy in OCD. Another study demonstrated that higher glucose metabolism in the OFC was associated with greater improvement with behavioral therapy and a worse outcome with fluoxetine treatment.[149]

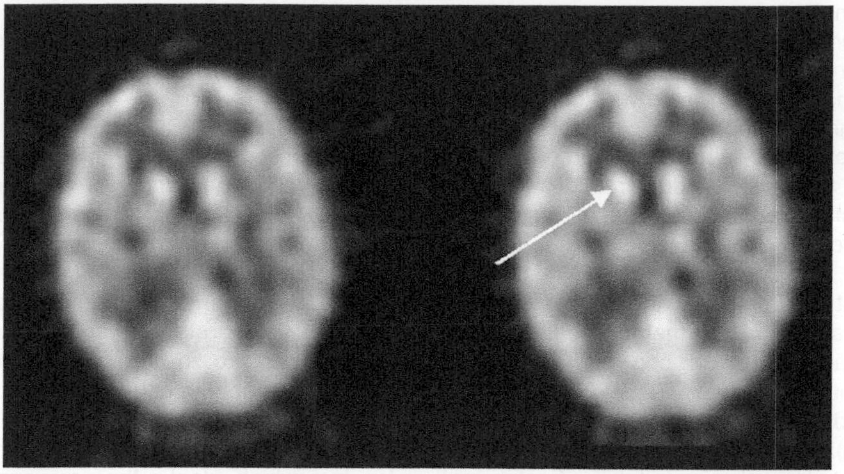

Fig. 5. FDG-PET of a patient with OCD showing increased glucose metabolism in the caudate nuclei bilaterally (*arrow*).

Behavior therapy responders also had significant bilateral decreases in caudate metabolism.[150] Furthermore, patients who responded to paroxetine had significantly lower metabolic rates in the right anterolateral OFC and right caudate nucleus and lower pretreatment metabolism in the left and right OFC predicted greater improvement with treatment.[151] These results suggest that subjects with differing patterns of metabolism preferentially respond to behavioral therapy versus medication. In patients with OCD, behavioral therapy responders have been shown to have significant bilateral decreases in caudate glucose metabolic rates compared with poor responders.[150] This study, as well as others, also suggests that there is a prefrontal cortico-striato-thalamic network that mediates the symptoms of OCD.[152] Neuroimaging studies have also revealed important findings in OCD. A study that used ^{11}C-MDL found a significant reduction of serotonin type 2A receptor availability in the frontal polar, dorsolateral, and medial frontal cortex as well as in the temporoparietal association cortex in OCD patients.[153] There was also a significant correlation between serotonin type 2A receptor availability in the OFC and dorsolateral frontal cortex and clinical severity of OCD. In addition, this same study used ^{11}C-raclopride PET and found a significant reduction of uptake in the whole striatum, possibly reflecting endogenous dopaminergic hyperactivity. Furthermore, the reduction in ^{11}C-raclopride binding is improved by treatment with fluvoxamine with concomitant improvement in symptoms.[154] Another study showed that OCD was associated with decreased serotonin transporter binding in the insular cortex as measured by ^{11}C-DASB PET imaging.[155] This finding suggests the potential role of the serotonergic system in the pathophysiology of OCD.

ALCOHOLISM

Studies of alcoholic patients with PET have generally found decreased whole-brain metabolic activity.[156,157] A study by Wik and colleagues[158] used CT and FDG–PET to examine patients with alcoholism. They found that alcoholic patients had reductions of 20% to 30% in cortical and subcortical brain regional metabolism compared with controls. Although the hypometabolism was diffusely distributed, the parietal areas were disproportionately affected. Other studies have reported frontal lobe hypometabolism. Also, studies have reported metabolic deficits in the left hemisphere more often than in the right.[159] A recent study suggests that there may be differences in the cerebral metabolism in women with alcoholism compared with men because women had less of a decrease in metabolism compared with men.[160] Patients with chronic alcoholism and cerebellar degeneration had significantly reduced glucose metabolism in the superior vermis compared with controls.[161] Volkow and colleagues[162] reported that the decrease in metabolism in chronic alcoholics correlated with the time since they last consumed alcohol. There were decreases in frontal and parietal metabolism that did not follow this pattern, suggesting that these changes might be a long-term component of the effects of chronic alcoholism. Patients who remained abstinent or who had minimal alcohol during longitudinal follow-up, however, showed partial recovery of glucose metabolism in 2 of 3 divisions of the frontal lobes and improvement on neuropsychological tests of general cognitive and executive functioning, whereas the patients who relapsed had further declines in these areas.[163] Examining the metabolic changes associated with detoxification showed a significant increase in global and regional (primarily frontal lobe) measures predominantly within 16 to 30 days.[164] Additional follow-up did not demonstrate additional changes suggesting that the effects of detoxification occur in the first 30 days.

Another study compared the effects of acute alcohol ingestion on brain metabolism in a group of chronic alcoholics and controls.[165] Subjects in each group underwent FDG-PET studies at baseline and after the administration of ethanol (1 g per kg). The results showed hypometabolism, particularly in the occipital, prefrontal, and cerebellar cortices, after acute ingestion of alcohol. These areas also correspond to the areas of the highest density of benzodiazepine receptors, which may be clinically relevant because benzodiazepines are used for the treatment of alcohol withdrawal. Compared with controls, alcoholics had a more marked metabolic deficit after ethanol ingestion but had fewer clinical symptoms, suggesting a tolerance to alcohol.

Studies have also explored the effects of alcohol on various neurotransmitter systems within the brain. GABA-benzodiazepine receptor function is altered in alcoholics as demonstrated by decreased sensitivity to lorazepam administration in the thalamus, basal ganglia, OFC, and cerebellum and may account for the decreased sensitivity to the effects of alcohol and benzodiazepines in these subjects.[162,166] For example, studies have shown low dopamine D2 receptor densities and less conclusive changes in the dopamine transporter densities among late-onset alcoholics and low presynaptic DA function observed in the left caudate of 2 patients, suggesting that this stage of alcoholism may be a heterogeneous disorder.[167,168] One study reported reduced binding in the striatal monoaminergic presynaptic terminals in severe chronic alcoholic patients, suggesting that the damaging effects of severe chronic alcoholism on the central nervous system are more extensive than previously considered.[169] A comparison of alcoholics with controls with a serotoninergic challenge demonstrated activation of the basal ganglia circuits involving the orbital and prefrontal areas in controls but a blunted response among alcoholics.[170] In a related study of alcoholic patients on disulfiram, there was decreased cerebral glucose metabolism and decreased flumazenil influx and distribution volume in patients receiving disulfiram, suggesting that this drug may be an important factor in the functional imaging studies of alcoholic patients.[171]

COCAINE ABUSE

The use of cocaine has steadily increased over the past few decades and has reached an almost epidemic proportion. Cocaine is one of the most addictive and toxic abused drugs.[172] PET studies have the potential of elucidating the mechanisms of the effects and the addictive properties of cocaine.[173] Initial studies with ^{11}C cocaine showed maximal uptake in the basal ganglia.[174] This uptake was rapid, reaching peak concentration in 4 to 8 minutes after injection and a clearance half-life of 20 minutes. Preadministration of nomifensine, which blocks the presynaptic reuptake of dopamine and norepinephrine, was shown to block the uptake of cocaine in the basal ganglia in this study. Another study has shown that the euphoric effects of cocaine correspond directly to the concentration of the drug in the basal ganglia,[175] corroborating the findings of the PET scan results.

PET studies of brain metabolism studies (**Fig. 6**) have shown that acute administration of cocaine in chronic cocaine abusers results in decreased metabolism in the cortical and subcortical structures.[176] The extent of metabolic decrease correlated with the subjective evidence of the euphoria. In patients with chronic cocaine abuse, the duration since detoxification affects the cerebral glucose metabolism. Volkow and colleagues[177] showed decreased frontal activity 8 days to 2 months after last cocaine use (more extensive decrement in the left compared with the right hemisphere) in chronic abusers compared with controls. Another study[178] of the acute changes after withdrawal of the drug showed that 1 week after last cocaine use, these patients had hypermetabolism in the OFC and the basal ganglia compared with normal controls and those studied 1 month after last cocaine use. Furthermore, hypermetabolism in these regions correlated with the subjective craving for cocaine. A follow-up study also showed similar findings, particularly affecting the right hemisphere, but this study indicated that dopamine enhancement is not sufficient to increase metabolism in the frontal regions.[179] The predominant correlation of craving within the right but not the left brain region suggests laterality of the addiction response. A similar pattern has been reported in patients with OCD,[180] although it is not clear whether or not the ritualistic behavior in OCD is comparable with the addictive behavior of cocaine abusers. The OFC and basal ganglia, areas

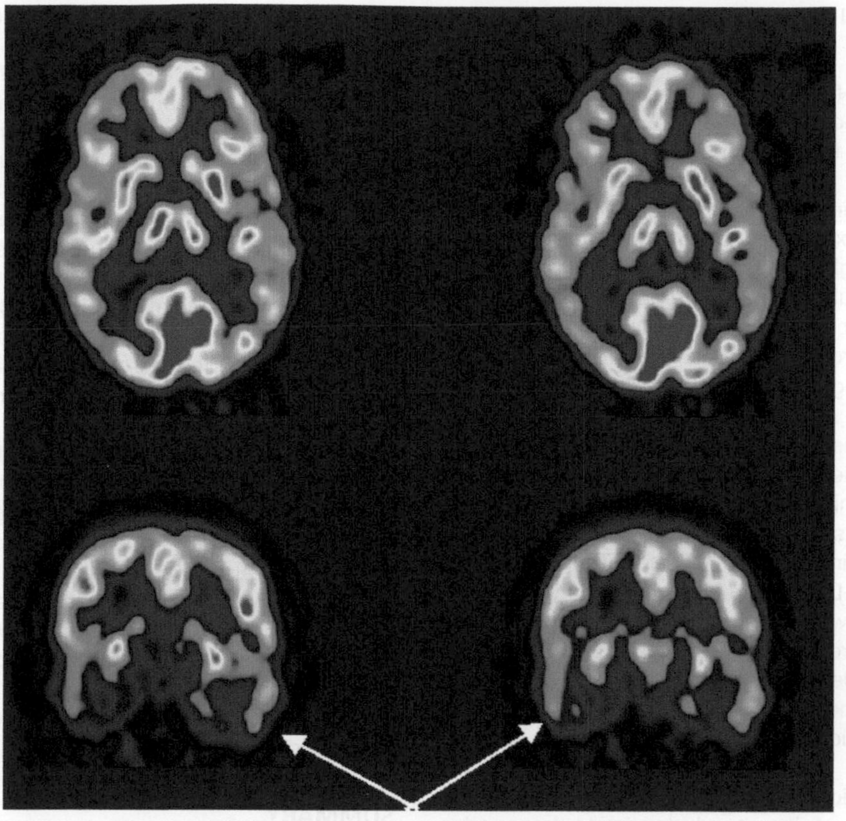

Fig. 6. FDG-PET scan of patient with chronic cocaine abuse showing global cortical decrease in glucose metabolism, particularly in the temporal lobes (*arrows*).

involved in cocaine abuse, however, are also involved in a circuit regulating repetitive behavior.[181] In terms of the actual craving for cocaine, one PET study showed a pattern of increased activity in limbic (amygdala and anterior cingulate) CBF and decreases in the basal ganglia while watching a video designed to induce craving[182] whereas another study showed activation of the temporal insula (involved with autonomic control) and the OFC (involved with expectancy and reinforcement) during a craving stimulus.[183]

PET receptor studies have attempted to determine the relationship between cocaine and dopamine receptors in the basal ganglia. For example, an ^{11}C-raclopride PET study showed modest decreases in D2 receptor availability throughout the striatum in chronic cocaine even though there was no clear relationship between D2 receptor availability and cocaine-induced cocaine-taking behavior.[184] Increased dopamine has been shown to play a role in cocaine's euphoric properties, and a decrease in dopamine presynaptic activity plays a role in withdrawal and possibly addictive properties.[185,186] Another study suggests that the thalamic dopamine pathways are also important in cocaine addiction.[187] A recent study suggests that low D1 receptor availability in the ventral striatum in cocaine abusers was associated with the choice to self-administer cocaine, suggesting that low D1 receptor availability may be associated with an increased risk of relapse.[188]

Cocaine has been shown to significantly block dopamine transporters.[189] The levels of blockade were comparable across several different routes of administration, including intravenous, intranasal, and smoked. Smoked cocaine induced significantly greater self-reports of a high than the other routes, likely due to the speed at which the cocaine is delivered to the brain, because there was no difference in the overall dopamine transporter blockade. Another study demonstrated that cocaine abusers have an enhanced sensitivity to lorazepam, suggesting a disruption of GABA pathways that may reflect, in part, cocaine withdrawal.[190] This same study noted that cocaine abusers also have intense sleepiness induced by lorazepam, suggesting potential clinical consequences of prescribing such medications to cocaine abusers.

ATTENTION-DEFICIT/HYPERACTIVITY DISORDER

Attention-deficit/hyperactivity disorder (ADHD) is characterized by inattention, hyperactivity, or impulsivity that produces impairment across a variety of cognitive, behavioral, and interpersonal domains. One of the first FDG-PET studies on ADHD examined 25 treatment-naive patients and found global cerebral glucose hypometabolism, particularly in the premotor cortex and in the superior PFC.[191] Two follow-up studies by the same group, however, did not find the same global or regional deficits.[192,193] Two other PET studies did suggest that there are frontostriatal abnormalities associated with ADHD.[194,195]

PET studies have shown that brain dopamine neurotransmission is disrupted in ADHD and that these deficits may underlie core symptoms of inattention and impulsivity.[196] One PET study showed lower L-^{11}C-DOPA use in adolescents with ADHD compared with control subjects, especially in subcortical regions.[197] ADHD may also be associated with deficits in the reward and motivation centers of the brain. Several studies have demonstrated reduced dopaminergic activity in patients with ADHD, particularly in the subcortical structures and midbrain.[198–200] Other studies, however, have reported increased dopamine transporter binding in the striatum of ADHD patients.[201] A PET study of 53 ADHD patients showed that specific binding of D2 receptors and dopamine transporters was lower in ADHD than in controls, particularly in regions of the dopamine reward pathway in the left side of the brain.[202] Ratings of attention correlated with D2/D3 receptor binding in the nucleus accumbens, midbrain, caudate, and hypothalamus and with dopamine transporter binding in the midbrain.

AUTISM

Autism is a neurodevelopmental disorder characterized by repetitive or obsessive interests and behavior as well as deficits in sociability and communication. An FDG-PET study showed that patients with autism spectrum disorders had greater metabolism in the right caudate nucleus and lower glucose metabolic rates bilaterally in the ventral caudate, putamen, and thalamus.[203] These results suggest that there is a deficit in the anterior cingulate–ventral striatum–anterior thalamic pathway in autistic patients with autism spectrum disorders. A PET study with $^{15}O-H_2O$ demonstrated decreased CBF in the superior temporal lobe in autistic patients that also correlated with the severity of disease.[204] This corroborated previous studies that also demonstrated hypoperfusion in the bilateral temporal lobes.[205,206] Another study on the effects of SSRI treatment in autism showed that metabolic rates were significantly higher in the right anterior cingulate gyrus and the OFC after fluoxetine treatment.[207] In addition, patients with higher metabolic rates in the medial frontal region and anterior cingulate pretreatment were more likely to respond to fluoxetine.

The pathophysiology of autism is also postulated to be related to abnormalities of the serotoninergic and dopaminergic systems. The actual pathophysiology of autism, however, remains to be fully elucidated. A recent study showed that serotonin transporter binding is significantly lower in the brain of autistic individuals compared with controls.[208] The decrease in the cingulate cortex was correlated with impairment of social cognition. There also was a significant correlation between repetitive or obsessive behaviors and the reduction of serotonin transporter binding in the thalamus. In the same group of autistic patients, dopamine transporter binding was significantly higher in the OFC and binding was inversely correlated with serotonin transporter binding.

SUMMARY

PET imaging has been used to assess a wide variety of psychiatric disorders. Most of these imaging results still lie in the realm of research, helping to understand the pathophysiology of different disorders, explore diagnostic criteria, and evaluate the effects of treatment. Future studies are needed to explore how the growing number of neurotransmitter ligands can be used in the study of psychiatric disorders. Ultimately, identifying and validating clinical applications will be necessary so that PET imaging continues to play a key role in the management of psychiatric disorders.

REFERENCES

1. Fu CHY, McGuire PK. Functional neuroimaging in psychiatry. Philos Trans R Soc Lond, B. Biol Sci 1999;354:1359–70.
2. Kung HF. Overview of radiopharmaceuticals for diagnosis of central nervous disorders. Crit Rev Clin Lab Sci 1991;28:269–86.
3. Maziere B, Maziere M. Positron emission tomography studies of brain receptors. Fundam Clin Pharmacol 1991;5:61–91.
4. Gatley SJ, DeGrado TR, Kornguth ML, et al. Radiopharmaceuticals for positron emission tomography: development of new, innovative tracers for

measuring the rates of physiologic and biochemical processes. Acta Radiol Suppl (Stockh) 1990; 374:7–11.
5. Kopin TJ. In-vivo quantitative imaging of catecholaminergic nerve terminals in brain and peripheral organs using positron emission tomography (PET). J Neural Transm Suppl 1990; 32:19–27.
6. Sadzot B, Mayberg HS, Frost JJ. Detection and quantification of opiate receptors in man by positron emission tomography. Potential applications to the study of pain. Neurophysiol Clin 1990;20:323–34.
7. Frost JJ. Receptor imaging by positron emission tomography and single-photon emission computed tomography. Invest Radiol 1992;27(Suppl 2):S54–8.
8. Abadie P, Baron JC, Bisserbe JG, et al. Central benzodiazepine receptors in human brain: estimation of regional Bmax and KD values with positron emission tomography. Eur J Pharmacol 1992;213: 107–15.
9. Varastet M, Brouillet E, Chavoix C, et al. In vivo visualization of central muscarinic receptors using [11C] quinuclidinyl benzilate and positron emission tomography in baboons. Eur J Pharmacol 1992; 213:275–84.
10. O'Connell RA, Van Heertum RL, Holt AR, et al. Single photon emission computed tomography in psychiatry. Clin Nucl Med 1987;12(Suppl 9):13.
11. Phelps ME, Mazziotta JC, Baxter L, et al. Positron emission tomographic study of affective disorders. Problems and strategies. Ann Neurol 1984; 15(Suppl):S149–56.
12. Bench CJ, Friston KJ, Brown RG, et al. The anatomy of melancholia—focal abnormalities of cerebral blood flow in major depression. Psychiatry Med 1992;22:607–15.
13. Dolan RJ, Bench CJ, Brown RG, et al. Regional cerebral blood flow abnormalities in depressed patients with cognitive impairment. J Neurol Neurosurg Psychiatr 1992;55:768–73.
14. Drevets WC, Price JL, Simpson JR Jr, et al. Subgenual prefrontal cortex abnormalities in mood disorders. Nature 1997;386(6627):824–7.
15. Ho AP, Gillin JC, Buchsbaum MS, et al. Brain glucose metabolism during non-rapid eye movement sleep in major depression. A positron emission tomography study. Arch Gen Psychiatry 1996;53(7):645–52.
16. Kumar A, Newberg A, Alavi A, et al. Regional cerebral glucose metabolism in late life depression and Alzheimer's disease: a preliminary positron emission tomography study. Proc Natl Acad Sci U S A 1993;90:7019–23.
17. Osuch EA, Ketter TA, Kimbrell TA, et al. Regional cerebral metabolism associated with anxiety symptoms in affective disorder patients. Biol Psychiatry 2000;48(10):1020–3.
18. Brody AL, Saxena S, Silverman DH, et al. Brain metabolic changes in major depressive disorder from pre- to post-treatment with paroxetine. Psychiatry Res 1999;91(3):127–39.
19. Milak MS, Parsey RV, Lee L, et al. Pretreatment regional brain glucose uptake in the midbrain on PET may predict remission from a major depressive episode after three months of treatment. Psychiatry Res 2009;173(1):63–70.
20. Konarski JZ, Kennedy SH, Segal ZV, et al. Predictors of nonresponse to cognitive behavioural therapy or venlafaxine using glucose metabolism in major depressive disorder. J Psychiatry Neurosci 2009;34(3):175–80.
21. Mayberg HS, Brannan SK, Tekell JL, et al. Regional metabolic effects of fluoxetine in major depression: serial changes and relationship to clinical response. Biol Psychiatry 2000;48(8):830–43.
22. Wu J, Buchsbaum MS, Gillin JC, et al. Prediction of antidepressant effects of sleep deprivation by metabolic rates in the ventral anterior cingulate and medial prefrontal cortex. Am J Psychiatry 1999;156(8):1149–58.
23. Smith GS, Reynolds CF 3rd, Pollock B, et al. Cerebral glucose metabolic response to combined total sleep deprivation and antidepressant treatment in geriatric depression. Am J Psychiatry 1999; 156(5):683–9.
24. Bewernick BH, Hurlemann R, Matusch A, et al. Nucleus accumbens deep brain stimulation decreases ratings of depression and anxiety in treatment-resistant depression. Biol Psychiatry 2010;67(2):110–6.
25. Baxter LR, Phelps ME, Mazziotta JC, et al. Cerebral metabolic rates for glucose in mood disorders. Arch Gen Psychiatry 1985;42:441–7.
26. Schwartz JM, Baxter LR, Mazziotta JC, et al. The differential diagnosis of depression. Relevance of positron emission tomography studies of cerebral glucose metabolism to the bipolar-unipolar dichotomy. JAMA 1987;258:1368–74.
27. Buchsbaum M, Wu J, Haier R, et al. Positron emission tomography assessment of effects of benzodiazepines on regional glucose metabolic rate in patients with anxiety disorder. Life Sci 1986;40: 2393–400.
28. Morris P, Rapoport GI. Neuroimaging and affective disorder in late life: a review. Can J Psychiatry 1990;35:347–54.
29. Meltzer CC, Price JC, Mathis CA, et al. PET imaging of serotonin type 2A receptors in late-life neuropsychiatric disorders. Am J Psychiatry 1999;156(12):1871–8.
30. Yatham LN, Liddle PF, Shiah IS, et al. Brain serotonin receptors in major depression: a positron emission tomography study. Arch Gen Psychiatry 2000;57(9):850–8.

31. Drevets WC, Frank E, Price JC, et al. Serotonin type-1A receptor imaging in depression. Nucl Med Biol 2000;27(5):499–507.
32. Drevets WC, Thase ME, Moses-Kolko EL, et al. Serotonin-1A receptor imaging in recurrent depression: replication and literature review. Nucl Med Biol 2007;34(7):865–77.
33. Biver F, Wikler D, Lotstra F, et al. Serotonin 5-HT2 receptor imaging in major depression: focal changes in orbito-insular cortex. Br J Psychiatry 1997;171:444–8.
34. Meyer JH. Imaging the serotonin transporter during major depressive disorder and antidepressant treatment. J Psychiatry Neurosci 2007;32: 86–102.
35. Zanardi R, Artigas F, Moresco R, et al. Increased 5-hydroxytryptamine-2 receptor binding in the frontal cortex of depressed patients responding to paroxetine treatment: a positron emission tomography scan study. J Clin Psychopharmacol 2001;21(1): 53–8.
36. Meyer JH, Kapur S, Eisfeld B, et al. The effect of paroxetine on 5-HT(2A) receptors in depression: an [(18)F]setoperone PET imaging study. Am J Psychiatry 2001;158(1):78–85.
37. Sargent PA, Kjaer KH, Bench CJ, et al. Brain serotonin1A receptor binding measured by positron emission tomography with [11C]WAY-100635: effects of depression and antidepressant treatment. Arch Gen Psychiatry 2000;57(2):174–80.
38. Saijo T, Takano A, Suhara T, et al. Effect of electroconvulsive therapy on 5-HT1A receptor binding in patients with depression: a PET study with [11C]WAY 100635. Int J Neuropsychopharmacology 2010;1–7. [Epub ahead of print].
39. Yatham LN, Liddle PF, Dennie J, et al. Decrease in brain serotonin 2 receptor binding in patients with major depression following desipramine treatment: a positron emission tomography study with fluorine-18-labeled setoperone. Arch Gen Psychiatry 1999;56(8):705–11.
40. Selvaraj S, Venkatesha Murthy N, Bhagwagar Z, et al. Diminished brain 5-HT transporter binding in major depression: a positron emission tomography study with [(11)C]DASB. Psychopharmacology (Berl) 2009. [Epub ahead of print].
41. Martinot M, Bragulat V, Artiges E, et al. Decreased presynaptic dopamine function in the left caudate of depressed patients with affective flattening and psychomotor retardation. Am J Psychiatry 2001; 158(2):314–6.
42. Saijo T, Takano A, Suhara T, et al. Electroconvulsive therapy decreases dopamine D(2) receptor binding in the anterior cingulate in patients with depression: a controlled study using positron emission tomography with radioligand [(11)C]FLB 457. J Clin Psychiatry 2009. [Epub ahead of print].
43. Pearlson GD, Wong DF, Tune LE, et al. In vivo D2 dopamine receptor density in psychotic and nonpsychotic patients with bipolar disorder. Arch Gen Psychiatry 1995;52(6):471–7.
44. Klumpers UM, Veltman DJ, Drent ML, et al. Reduced parahippocampal and lateral temporal GABAA-[11C]flumazenil binding in major depression: preliminary results. J Nucl Med Mol Imaging 2010;37(3):565–74.
45. Reiman E, Rachle M, Butler F, et al. A focal brain abnormality in panic disorder: a severe form of anxiety. Nature 1984;310:683–5.
46. Reiman E, Rachle M, Robbins E, et al. Neuroanatomical correlates of a lactate-induced anxiety attack. Arch Gen Psychiatry 1989;46:493–500.
47. Reiman E, Rachle M, Robbins E, et al. The application of positron emission tomography to the study of panic disorder. Am J Psychiatry 1986; 143:469–77.
48. Wu JC, Buchsbaum MS, Hershey TG, et al. PET in generalized anxiety disorder. Biol Psychiatry 1991; 29(12):1181–99.
49. Kern S, Oakes TR, Stone CK, et al. Glucose metabolic changes in the prefrontal cortex are associated with HPA axis response to a psychosocial stressor. Psychoneuroendocrinology 2008;33(4): 517–29.
50. Mountz J, Modell J, Wilson M, et al. PET evaluation of cerebral blood flow during anxiety state in simple phobia. Arch Gen Psychiatry 1989;46:501–4.
51. Pardo JV, Fox PT, Raichle ME. Localization of a human system for sustained attention by positron emission tomography. Nature 1991;349:61–4.
52. Herzog H, Lele VR, Kuwert T, et al. Changed pattern of regional glucose metabolism during Yoga meditative relaxation. Neuropsychobiology 1990-1991;23:182–7.
53. Lou HC, Kjaer TW, Friberg L, et al. A $^{15}O-H_2O$ PET study of meditation and the resting state of normal consciousness. Hum Brain Mapp 1999;7:98–105.
54. Newberg AB, Iversen J. The neural basis of the complex mental task of meditation: neurotransmitter and neurochemical considerations. Med Hypotheses 2003;61(2):282–91.
55. Akimova E, Lanzenberger R, Kasper S. The serotonin-1A receptor in anxiety disorders. Biol Psychiatry 2009;66(7):627–35.
56. Kjaer TW, Bertelsen C, Piccini P, et al. Increased dopamine tone during meditation-induced change of consciousness. Brain Res Cogn Brain Res 2002; 13(2):255–9.
57. Pruessner JC, Dedovic K, Pruessner M, et al. Stress regulation in the central nervous system: evidence from structural and functional neuroimaging studies in human populations—2008 Curt Richter Award Winner. Psychoneuroendocrinology 2010;35(1):179–91.

58. Fernandez M, Pissiota A, Frans O, et al. Brain function in a patient with torture related post-traumatic stress disorder before and after fluoxetine treatment: a positron emission tomography provocation study. Neurosci Lett 2001;297(2):101–14.
59. Molina ME, Isoardi R, Prado MN, et al. Basal cerebral glucose distribution in long-term post-traumatic stress disorder. World J Biol Psychiatry 2007(Sep 13);1–9.
60. Shin LM, McNally RJ, Kosslyn SM, et al. Regional cerebral blood flow during script-driven imagery in childhood sexual abuse-related PTSD: a PET investigation. Am J Psychiatry 1999;156(4):575–84.
61. Shin LM, Orr SP, Carson MA, et al. Regional cerebral blood flow in the amygdala and medial prefrontal cortex during traumatic imagery in male and female Vietnam veterans with PTSD. Arch Gen Psychiatry 2004;61(2):168–76.
62. Semple WE, Goyer PF, McCormick R, et al. Higher brain blood flow at amygdala and lower frontal cortex blood flow in PTSD patients with comorbid cocaine and alcohol abuse compared with normals. Psychiatr 2000;63(1):65–74.
63. Liddle PF. PET scanning and schizophrenia—what progress? Psychiatry Med 1992;22:557–60.
64. Sedvall G. The current status of PET scanning with respect to schizophrenia. Neuropsychopharmacology 1992;7:41–54.
65. Cleghorn JM, Zipursky RB, List SJ. Structural and functional brain imaging in schizophrenia. J Psychiatry Neurosci 1991;16:53–74.
66. Kim JJ, Mohamed S, Andreasen NC, et al. Regional neural dysfunctions in chronic schizophrenia studied with positron emission tomography. Am J Psychiatry 2000;157(4):542–8.
67. Ingvar DH, Franzen G. Abnormalities of cerebral blood flow distribution in patients with chronic schizophrenia. Acta Psychiatr Scand 1974;50:425–62.
68. Andreasen NC, O'Leary DS, Flaum M, et al. Hypofrontality in schizophrenia: distributed dysfunctional circuits in neuroleptic-naive patients. Lancet 1997;349(9067):1730–4.
69. Lehrer DS, Christian BT, Mantil J, et al. Thalamic and prefrontal FDG uptake in never medicated patients with schizophrenia. Am J Psychiatry 2005;162(5):931–8.
70. Gur RE, Resnick SM, Alavi A, et al. Regional brain function in schizophrenia I. A positron emission tomography study. Arch Gen Psychiatry 1987;44:119–25.
71. Wiesel FA, Wik G, Sjogren I, et al. Altered relationships between metabolic rates of glucose in brain regions of schizophrenic patients. Acta Psychiatr Scand 1987;76:642–7.
72. Wiesel FA, Wik G, Sjogren I, et al. Regional brain glucose metabolism in drug-free schizophrenic patients and clinical correlates. Acta Psychiatr Scand 1987;76:628–41.
73. Soyka M, Koch W, Möller HJ, et al. Hypermetabolic pattern in frontal cortex and other brain regions in unmedicated schizophrenia patients. Results from a FDG-PET study. Eur Arch Psychiatry Clin Neurosci 2005;255(5):308–12.
74. Volkow ND, Wolf AP, Van Gelder P, et al. Phenomenological correlates of metabolic activity in 18 patients with chronic schizophrenia. Am J Psychiatry 1987;144:151–8.
75. McGuire PK, Quested DJ, Spence SA, et al. Pathophysiology of 'positive' thought disorder in schizophrenia. Br J Psychiatry 1998;173:231–5.
76. Buchanan RW, Breier A, Kirkpatrick B, et al. The deficit syndrome. Functional and structural characteristics. Schizoprenia Res 1991;4:400–1.
77. Schroder J, Buchsbaum MS, Siegel BV, et al. Cerebral metabolic activity correlates of subsyndromes in chronic schizophrenia. Schizophr Res 1996;19(1):41–53.
78. Liddle PF, Friston KJ, Frith CD, et al. Cerebral blood flow and mental processes in schizophrenia. J R Soc Med 1992;85:224–7.
79. Liddle PF, Friston KJ, Frith CD, et al. Patterns of cerebral blood flow in schizophrenia. Br J Psychol 1992;160:179–86.
80. Spence SA, Hirsch SR, Brooks DJ, et al. Prefrontal cortex activity in people with schizophrenia and control subjects. Evidence from positron emission tomography for remission of 'hypofrontality' with recovery from acute schizophrenia. Br J Psychiatry 1998;172:316–23.
81. Sabri O, Erkwoh R, Schreckenberger M, et al. Correlation of positive symptoms exclusively to hyperperfusion or hypoperfusion of cerebral cortex in never-treated schizophrenics. Lancet 1997;349(9067):1735–9.
82. Haznedar MM, Buchsbaum MS, Luu C, et al. Decreased anterior cingulate gyrus metabolic rate in schizophrenia. Am J Psychiatry 1997;154(5):682–4.
83. Fujimoto T, Takeuch K, Matsumoto T, et al. Abnormal glucose metabolism in the anterior cingulate cortex in patients with schizophrenia. Psychiatry Res 2007;154(1):49–58.
84. Hazlett EA, Buchsbaum MS, Byne W, et al. Three-dimensional analysis with MRI and PET of the size, shape, and function of the thalamus in the schizophrenia spectrum. Am J Psychiatry 1999;156(8):1190–9.
85. Buchsbaum MS, Someya T, Teng CY, et al. PET and MRI of the thalamus in never-medicated patients with schizophrenia. Am J Psychiatry 1996;153(2):191–9.
86. Katz M, Buchsbaum MS, Siegel BV Jr, et al. Correlational patterns of cerebral glucose metabolism in

never-medicated schizophrenics. Neuropsychobiology 1996;33(1):1–11.
87. Siegel BV Jr, Buchsbaum MS, Bunney WE Jr, et al. Cortical-striatal-thalamic circuits and brain glucose metabolic activity in 70 unmedicated male schizophrenic patients. Am J Psychiatry 1993;150(9): 1325–36.
88. Gur RE, Chin S. Laterality in functional brain imaging studies of schizophrenia. Schizophr Bull 1999;25(1):141–56.
89. Gur RE, Resnick SM, Gur RC, et al. Regional brain function in schizophrenia. II. Repeated evaluation with positron emission tomography. Arch Gen Psychiatry 1987;44:126–9.
90. Gur RE, Resnick SM, Gur RC. Laterality and frontality of cerebral blood flow and metabolism in schizophrenia. Relationship to symptom specificity. Psychiatry Res 1989;27:325–34.
91. Sheppard G, Gruzelier J, Manchanda R, et al. Positron emission tomographic scanning in predominantly never-treated acute schizophrenic patients. Lancet 1983;2:1448–52.
92. Early TS, Reiman EM, Raichle ME, et al. Left globus pallidus abnormality in never-medicated patients with schizophrenia. Proc Natl Acad Sci U S A 1987;84:561–3.
93. Laakso A, Vilkman H, Alakare B, et al. Striatal dopamine transporter binding in neuroleptic-naive patients with schizophrenia studied with positron emission tomography. Am J Psychiatry 2000; 157(2):269–71.
94. Cohen RM, Semple WE, Gross M, et al. From syndrome to illness. Delineating the pathophysiology of schizophrenia with PET. Schizophr Bull 1988;14:169–76.
95. Cohen RM, Semple WE, Gross M, et al. Dysfunction in a prefrontal substrate of sustained attention in schizophrenia. Life Sci 1987;43:2031–9.
96. DeLisi LE, Buchsbaum MS, Holcomb HH, et al. Increased temporal lobe glucose use in chronic schizophrenic patients. Biol Psychiatry 1989;25: 835–51.
97. Gunther W. MRI-SPECT and PET-EEG findings on brain dysfunction in schizophrenia. Prog Neuropsychopharmacol Biol Psychiatry 1992;16:445–62.
98. Siegel BV Jr, Nuechterlein KH, Abel L, et al. Glucose metabolic correlates of continuous performance test performance in adults with a history of infantile autism, schizophrenics, and controls. Schizophr Res 1995;17(1):85–94.
99. Carter CS, Mintun M, Nichols T, et al. Anterior cingulate gyrus dysfunction and selective attention deficits in schizophrenia: [15O]H2O PET study during single-trial Stroop task performance. Am J Psychiatry 1997;154(12):1670–5.
100. Artiges E, Martinot JL, Verdys M, et al. Altered hemispheric functional dominance during word generation in negative schizophrenia. Schizophr Bull 2000;26(3):709–21.
101. Heckers S, Curran T, Goff D, et al. Abnormalities in the thalamus and prefrontal cortex during episodic object recognition in schizophrenia. Biol Psychiatry 2000;48(7):651–7.
102. Crespo-Facorro B, Paradiso S, Andreasen NC, et al. Recalling word lists reveals "cognitive dysmetria" in schizophrenia: a positron emission tomography study. Am J Psychiatry 1999;156(3):386–92.
103. Heckers S, Goff D, Schacter DL, et al. Functional imaging of memory retrieval in deficit vs nondeficit schizophrenia. Arch Gen Psychiatry 1999;56(12): 1117–23.
104. Carter CS, Perlstein W, Ganguli R, et al. Functional hypofrontality and working memory dysfunction in schizophrenia. Am J Psychiatry 1998;155(9): 1285–7.
105. Volkow ND, Wolf AP, Brodie JD, et al. Brain interactions in chronic schizophrenics under resting and activation conditions. Schizophr Res 1988;1:47–53.
106. Andreasen NC, O'Leary DS, Cizadlo T, et al. Schizophrenia and cognitive dysmetria: a positron-emission tomography study of dysfunctional prefrontal-thalamic-cerebellar circuitry. PNAS 1996;93(18):9985–90.
107. Artiges E, Salame P, Recasens C, et al. Working memory control in patients with schizophrenia: a PET study during a random number generation task. Am J Psychiatry 2000;157(9):1517–9.
108. Heckers S, Rauch SL, Goff D, et al. Impaired recruitment of the hippocampus during conscious recollection in schizophrenia. Nat Neurosci 1998; 1(4):318–23.
109. Fletcher PC, McKenna PJ, Frith CD, et al. Brain activations in schizophrenia during a graded memory task studied with functional neuroimaging. Arch Gen Psychiatry 1998;55(11):1001–8.
110. Ragland JD, Gur RC, Glahn DC, et al. Frontotemporal cerebral blood flow change during executive and declarative memory tasks in schizophrenia: a positron emission tomography study. Neuropsychology 1998;12(3):399–413.
111. Hyde TM, Weinberger DR. The brain in schizophrenia. Semin Neurol 1990;10:275–85.
112. Sedvall G. Monoamines and schizophrenia. Acta Psychiatr Scand Suppl 1990;358:7–13.
113. Okubo Y, Suhara T, Suzuki K, et al. Decreased prefrontal dopamine D1 receptors in schizophrenia revealed by PET. Nature 1997;385(6617):634–6.
114. Sedvall G, Farde L, Hall H, et al. PET scanning—a new tool in clinical psychopharmacology. Psychiatr Serv 1988;5:27–33.
115. Farde L, Nordstrom AL, Eriksson L, et al. Comparison of methods used with (11C)NMSP for the PET-determination of central D2 dopamine receptors. Clin Neuropharmacol 1990;13:87–8.

116. Wong DF, Wagner HN Jr, Tune LE, et al. Positron emission tomography reveals elevated D2 dopamine receptors in drug-naive schizophrenics. Science 1986;234:1558–63.
117. Tune L, Barta P, Wong D, et al. Striatal dopamine D2 receptor quantification and superior temporal gyrus: volume determination in 14 chronic schizophrenic subjects. Psychiatry Res 1996;67(2):155–8.
118. Seeman P, Guan HC, Niznik HB. Endogenous dopamine lowers the dopamine D2 receptor density as measured by (3H)raclopride: implications for positron emission tomography of the human brain. Synapse 1989;3:96–7.
119. Kessler RM, Woodward ND, Riccardi P, et al. Dopamine D2 receptor levels in striatum, thalamus, substantia nigra, limbic regions, and cortex in schizophrenic subjects. Biol Psychiatry 2009; 65(12):1024–31.
120. Howes OD, Montgomery AJ, Asselin MC, et al. Molecular imaging studies of the striatal dopaminergic system in psychosis and predictions for the prodromal phase of psychosis. Br J Psychiatry Suppl 2007;51:s13–8.
121. Howes OD, Montgomery AJ, Asselin MC, et al. Elevated striatal dopamine function linked to prodromal signs of schizophrenia. Arch Gen Psychiatry 2009;66(1):13–20.
122. Hietala J, Syvalahti E, Vilkman H, et al. Depressive symptoms and presynaptic dopamine function in neuroleptic-naive schizophrenia. Schizophr Res 1999;35(1):41–50.
123. Verhoeff NP, Meyer JH, Kecojevic A, et al. A voxel-by-voxel analysis of [18F]setoperone PET data shows no substantial serotonin 5-HT(2A) receptor changes in schizophrenia. Psychiatry Res 2000; 99(3):123–35.
124. Okubo Y, Suhara T, Suzuki K, et al. Serotonin 5-HT2 receptors in schizophrenic patients studied by positron emission tomography. Life Sci 2000; 66(25):2455–64.
125. Ngan ET, Yatham LN, Ruth TJ, et al. Decreased serotonin 2A receptor densities in neuroleptic-naive patients with schizophrenia: a PET study using [(18)F]setoperone. Am J Psychiatry 2000; 157(6):1016–8.
126. Volkow ND, Brodie JD, Wolf AP, et al. Brain metabolism in patients with schizophrenia before and after acute neuroleptic administration. J Neurol Neurosurg Psychiatr 1986;49:1199–202.
127. Resnick SM, Gur RE, Alavi A, et al. Positron emission tomography and subcortical glucose metabolism in schizophrenia. Psychiatry Res 1988;24:1–11.
128. Buchsbaum MS, Potkin SG, Siegel BV Jr, et al. Striatal metabolic rate and clinical response to neuroleptics in schizophrenia. Arch Gen Psychiatry 1992;49(12):966–74.
129. Bartlett EJ, Brodie JD, Simkowitz P, et al. Effect of a haloperidol challenge on regional brain metabolism in neuroleptic-responsive and nonresponsive schizophrenic patients. Am J Psychiatry 1998; 155(3):337–43.
130. Kapur S, Zipursky R, Jones C, et al. Relationship between dopamine D(2) occupancy, clinical response, and side effects: a double-blind PET study of first-episode schizophrenia. Am J Psychiatry 2000;157(4):514–20.
131. Farde L, Wiesel FA, Halldin C, et al. Central D2-dopamine receptor occupancy in schizophrenic patients treated with antipsychotic drugs. Arch Gen Psychiatry 1988;45:71–6.
132. Kapur S, Remington G, Jones C, et al. High levels of dopamine D2 receptor occupancy with low-dose haloperidol treatment: a PET study. Am J Psychiatry 1996;153(7):948–50.
133. Miller DD, Andreasen NC, O'Leary DS, et al. Effect of antipsychotics on regional cerebral blood flow measured with positron emission tomography. Neuropsychopharmacology 1997;17(4):230–40.
134. Wolkin A, Barouche F, Wolf AP, et al. Dopamine blockade and clinical response. Evidence for two biological subgroups of schizophrenia. Am J Psychiatry 1989;146:905–8.
135. Martinot JL, Pailliere-Martinot ML, Loc HC, et al. Central D2 receptor blockade and antipsychotic effects of neuroleptics. Preliminary study with positron emission tomography. Psychiatr Psychiatrobiol 1990;5:231–40.
136. Sedvall G, Farde L, Stone-Lander S, et al. Dopamine D1-receptor binding in the living human brain. In: Breese GR, Creese I, editors. Neurobiology of central D1-dopamine receptors. New York: Plenum; 1986.
137. Farde L, Wiesel F-A, Nordstrom A-L, et al. D1 and D2-dopamine receptor occupancy during treatment with conventional and atypical neuroleptics. Psychiatropharmacol 1989;99:S28–31.
138. Kapur S, Zipursky R, Jones C, et al. A positron emission tomography study of quetiapine in schizophrenia: a preliminary finding of an antipsychotic effect with only transiently high dopamine D2 receptor occupancy. Arch Gen Psychiatry 2000;57(6):553–9.
139. Kessler RM, Ansari MS, Riccardi P, et al. Occupancy of striatal and extrastriatal dopamine D2 receptors by clozapine and quetiapine. Neuropsychopharmacology 2006;31(9):1991–2001 [Epub 2006 May 31].
140. Agid O, Mamo D, Ginovart N, et al. Striatal vs extrastriatal dopamine D2 receptors in antipsychotic response–a double-blind PET study in schizophrenia. Neuropsychopharmacology 2007;32(6): 1209–15.
141. Kapur S, Cho R, Jones C, et al. Is amoxapine an atypical antipsychotic? Positron-emission

tomography investigation of its dopamine2 and serotonin2 occupancy. Biol Psychiatry 1999;45(9): 1217–20.
142. Kapur S, Zipursky RB, Remington G, et al. 5-HT2 and D2 receptor occupancy of olanzapine in schizophrenia: a PET investigation. Am J Psychiatry 1998;155(7):921–8.
143. Cohen RM, Nordahl TE, Semple WE, et al. The brain metabolic patterns of clozapine- and fluphenazine-treated female patients with schizophrenia: evidence of a sex effect. Neuropsychopharmacology 1999;21(5):632–40.
144. Baxter L, Schwartz J, Mazziotta J, et al. Cerebral glucose metabolic rates in nondepressed patients with obsessive-compulsive disorder. Am J Psychiatry 1988;145:1560–3.
145. Nordahl TE, Benkelfat C, Semple W, et al. Cerebral glucose metabolic rates in obsessive compulsive disorder. Neuropsychopharmacology 1989;2:23–8.
146. Sawle GV, Hymas NF, Lees AJ, et al. Obsessional slowness. Functional studies with positron emission tomography. Brain 1991;114:2191–202.
147. Insel TR, Winslow JT. Neurobiology of obsessive-compulsive disorder. Psychiatr Clin North Am 1992;15:813–24.
148. Swedo SE, Schapiro MB, Grady CL, et al. Cerebral glucose metabolism in childhood-onset obsessive-compulsive disorder. Arch Gen Psychiatry 1989; 46:518–23.
149. Brody AL, Saxena S, Schwartz JM, et al. FDG-PET predictors of response to behavioral therapy and pharmacotherapy in obsessive compulsive disorder. Psychiatry Res 1998;84(1):1–6.
150. Schwartz JM, Stoessel PW, Baxter LR, et al. Systematic changes in cerebral glucose metabolic rate after successful behavior modification treatment of obsessive-compulsive disorder. Arch Gen Psychiatry 1996;53(2):109–13.
151. Saxena S, Brody AL, Maidment KM, et al. Localized orbitofrontal and subcortical metabolic changes and predictors of response to paroxetine treatment in obsessive-compulsive disorder. Neuropsychopharmacology 1999;21(6):683–93.
152. Rauch SL, Jenike MA, Alpert NM, et al. Regional cerebral blood flow measured during symptom provocation in obsessive-compulsive disorder using oxygen 15-labeled carbon dioxide and positron emission tomography. Arch Gen Psychiatry 1994;51(1):62–70.
153. Perani D, Garibotto V, Gorini A, et al. In vivo PET study of 5HT(2A) serotonin and D(2) dopamine dysfunction in drug-naive obsessive-compulsive disorder. Neuroimage 2008;42(1):306–14.
154. Moresco RM, Pietra L, Henin M, et al. Fluvoxamine treatment and D2 receptors: a pet study on OCD drug-naïve patients. Neuropsychopharmacology 2007;32(1):197–205.
155. Matsumoto R, Ichise M, Ito H, et al. Reduced serotonin transporter binding in the insular cortex in patients with obsessive-compulsive disorder: a [11C]DASB PET study. Neuroimage 2010;49(1): 121–6.
156. Samson Y, Baron JC, Feline A, et al. Local cerebral glucose utilization in chronic alcoholics, a positron tomography study. J Neurol Neurosurg Psychiatr 1986;49:1165–70.
157. Sach H, Russel JAG, Christman DR, et al. Alterations in regional cerebral glucose metabolic rate in non-Korsakoff chronic alcoholism. Arch Neurol 1987;44:1242–51.
158. Wik G, Borg S, Sjogren I, et al. Positron emission tomography determination of regional cerebral glucose metabolism in alcohol-dependent men and healthy controls using 11C-glucose. Acta Psychiatr Scand 1988;78:234–41.
159. Volkow ND, Fowler JS. Neuropsychiatric disorders. Investigation of schizophrenia and substance abuse. Semin Nucl Med 1992;22:254–67.
160. Wang GJ, Volkow ND, Fowler JS, et al. Regional cerebral metabolism in female alcoholics of moderate severity does not differ from that of controls. Alcohol Clin Exp Res 1998;22(8):1850–4.
161. Gilman S, Adams K, Koeppe RA, et al. Cerebellar hypometabolism in alcoholic cerebellar degeneration studied with FDG and PET. Neurol 1988;38:365.
162. Volkow ND, Wang G-J, Hitzemann R, et al. Decreased cerebral response to inhibitory neurotransmission in alcoholics. Am J Psychiatry 1993; 150:417–22.
163. Johnson-Greene D, Adams KM, Gilman S, et al. Effects of abstinence and relapse upon neuropsychological function and cerebral glucose metabolism in severe chronic alcoholism. J Clin Exp Neuropsychol 1997;19(3):378–85.
164. Volkow ND, Wang GJ, Hitzemann R, et al. Recovery of brain glucose metabolism in detoxified alcoholics. Am J Psychiatry 1994;151(2):178–83.
165. Volkow ND, Hitzemann R, Wolf AP, et al. Acute effects of ethanol on regional brain glucose metabolism and transport. Psychiatry Res 1990; 35:39–48.
166. Volkow ND, Wang GJ, Begleiter H, et al. Regional brain metabolic response to lorazepam in subjects at risk for alcoholism. Alcohol Clin Exp Res 1995; 19(2):510–6.
167. Volkow ND, Wang GJ, Fowler JS, et al. Decreases in dopamine receptors but not in dopamine transporters in alcoholics. Alcohol Clin Exp Res 1996; 20(9):1594–8.
168. Tiihonen J, Vilkman H, Rasanen P, et al. Striatal presynaptic dopamine function in type 1 alcoholics measured with positron emission tomography. Mol Psychiatry 1998;3(2):156–61.

169. Gilman S, Koeppe RA, Adams KM, et al. Decreased striatal monoaminergic terminals in severe chronic alcoholism demonstrated with (+)[11C]dihydrotetrabenazine and positron emission tomography. Ann Neurol 1998;44(3):326–33.
170. Hommer D, Andreasen P, Rio D, et al. Effects of m-chlorophenylpiperazine on regional brain glucose utilization: a positron emission tomographic comparison of alcoholic and control subjects. J Neurosci 1997;17(8):2796–806, 1997.
171. Gilman S, Adams KM, Johnson-Greene D, et al. Effects of disulfiram on positron emission tomography and neuropsychological studies in severe chronic alcoholism. Alcohol Clin Exp Res 1996; 20(8):1456–61.
172. Johanson CE, Fishman MW. The pharmacology of cocaine related to its abuse. Pharmacol Rev 1989;41:3–52.
173. Strickland TL, Miller BL, Kowell A, et al. Neurobiology of cocaine-induced organic brain impairment: contributions from functional neuroimaging. Neuropsychol Rev 1998;8(1):1–9.
174. Fowler JS, Volkow ND, Wolf AP, et al. Mapping cocaine binding sites in human and baboon brain in vivo. Synapse 1989;4:371–7.
175. Cook CE, Jeffcoat AR, Perez-Reys M. Pharmacokinetic studies of cocaine and phencyclidine in man. In: Barnett G, Chiang CN, editors. Pharmacokinetics and pharmacodynamics of psychoactive drugs. Foster City (CA): Biomedical Publications; 1985. p. 48–74.
176. London ED, Cascella NG, Wong DF, et al. Cocaine-induced reduction of glucose utilization in human brain. A study using positron emission tomography and (Fluorine-18)-fluorodeoxyglucose. Arch Gen Psychiatry 1990;47:567–74.
177. Volkow ND, Hitzemann R, Wang GJ, et al. Long-term frontal brain metabolic changes in cocaine abusers. Synapse 1992;11:184–90.
178. Volkow ND, Fowler JS, Wolf AP, et al. Changes in brain glucose metabolism in cocaine dependence and withdrawal. Am J Psychiatry 1991;148:621–6.
179. Volkow ND, Wang GJ, Fowler JS, et al. Association of methylphenidate-induced craving with changes in right striato-orbitofrontal metabolism in cocaine abusers: implications in addiction. Am J Psychiatry 1999;156(1):19–26.
180. Baxter L, Phelps M, Mazziotta J, et al. Local cerebral glucose metabolic rates in obsessive-compulsive disorder. A comparison with rates in unipolar depression and normal controls. Arch Gen Psychiatry 1987;44:211–8.
181. Modell JG, Mountz JM, Curtis G, et al. Neurophysiologic dysfunctions in basal ganglia limbic striatal and thalamorcortical circuit as a pathogenetic mechanism of obsessive compulsive disorder. J Neuropsychiatry 1989;1:27–36.
182. Childress AR, Mozley PD, McElgin W, et al. Limbic activation during cue-induced cocaine craving. Am J Psychiatry 1999;156(1):11–8.
183. Wang GJ, Volkow ND, Fowler JS, et al. Regional brain metabolic activation during craving elicited by recall of previous drug experiences. Life Sci 1999;64(9):775–84.
184. Martinez D, Broft A, Foltin RW, et al. Cocaine dependence and d2 receptor availability in the functional subdivisions of the striatum: relationship with cocaine-seeking behavior. Neuropsychopharmacol 2004;29(6):1190–202.
185. Schlaepfer TE, Pearlson GD, Wong DF, et al. PET study of competition between intravenous cocaine and [11C]raclopride at dopamine receptors in human subjects. Am J Psychiatry 1997;154(9): 1209–13.
186. Wu JC, Bell K, Najafi A, et al. Decreasing striatal 6-FDOPA uptake with increasing duration of cocaine withdrawal. Neuropsychopharmacology 1997; 17(6):402–9.
187. Volkow ND, Wang GJ, Fowler JS, et al. Decreased striatal dopaminergic responsiveness in detoxified cocaine-dependent subjects. Nature 1997; 386(6627):830–3.
188. Martinez D, Slifstein M, Narendran R, et al. Dopamine D1 receptors in cocaine dependence measured with PET and the choice to self-administer cocaine. Neuropsychopharmacol 2009;34(7): 1774–82.
189. Volkow ND, Wang GJ, Fischman MW, et al. Effects of route of administration on cocaine induced dopamine transporter blockade in the human brain. Life Sci 2000;67(12):1507–15.
190. Volkow ND, Wang GJ, Fowler JS, et al. Enhanced sensitivity to benzodiazepines in active cocaine-abusing subjects: a PET study. Am J Psychiatry 1998;155(2):200–6.
191. Zametkin AJ, Nordahl TE, Gross M, et al. Cerebral glucose metabolism in adults with hyperactivity of childhood onset. N Engl J Med 1990; 20:1361–6.
192. Ernst M, Libenauer LL, King AC, et al. Reduced brain metabolism in hyperactive girls. J Am Acad Child Adolesc Psychiatry 1994;33:858–68.
193. Zametkin AJ, Liebenauer LL, Fitzgerald GA, et al. Brain metabolism in teenagers with attention-deficit hyperactivity disorder. Arch Gen Psychiatry 1993; 50:333–40.
194. Ernst M, Grant SJ, London ED, et al. Decision making in adolescents with behavior disorders and adults with substance abuse. Am J Psychiatry 2003;160:33–40.
195. Schweitzer JB, Faber TL, Grafton ST, et al. Alterations in the functional anatomy of working memory in adult attention deficit hyperactivity disorder. Am J Psychiatry 2000;157:278–80.

196. Rosa Neto P, Lou H, Cumming P, et al. Methylphenidate-evoked potentiation of extracellular dopamine in the brain of adolescents with premature birth. Ann N Y Acad Sci 2002;965:434–9.
197. Forssberg H, Fernell E, Waters S, et al. Altered pattern of brain dopamine synthesis in male adolescents with attention deficit hyperactivity disorder. Behav Brain Funct 2006;2:40.
198. Volkow ND, Wang GJ, Newcorn J, et al. Depressed dopamine activity in caudate and preliminary evidence of limbic involvement in adults with attention-deficit/hyperactivity disorder. Arch Gen Psychiatry 2007;64(8):932–40.
199. Volkow ND, Wang GJ, Newcorn J, et al. Brain dopamine transporter levels in treatment and drug naïve adults with ADHD. Neuroimage 2007;34(3):1182–90.
200. Jucaite A, Fernell E, Halldin C, et al. Reduced midbrain dopamine transporter binding in male adolescents with attention-deficit/hyperactivity disorder: association between striatal dopamine markers and motor hyperactivity. Biol Psychiatry 2005;57(3):229–38.
201. Spencer TJ, Biederman J, Madras BK, et al. Further evidence of dopamine transporter dysregulation in ADHD: a controlled PET imaging study using altropane. Biol Psychiatry 2007;62(9):1059–61.
202. Volkow ND, Wang GJ, Kollins SH, et al. Evaluating dopamine reward pathway in ADHD: clinical implications. JAMA 2009;302(10):1084–91.
203. Haznedar MM, Buchsbaum MS, Hazlett EA, et al. Volumetric analysis and three-dimensional glucose metabolic mapping of the striatum and thalamus in patients with autism spectrum disorders. Am J Psychiatry 2006;163(7):1252–63.
204. Gendry Meresse I, Zilbovicius M, Boddaert N, et al. Autism severity and temporal lobe functional abnormalities. Ann Neurol 2005;58(3):466–9.
205. Ohnishi T, Matsuda H, Hashimoto T, et al. Abnormal regional cerebral blood flow in childhood autism. Brain 2000;123:1838–44.
206. Zilbovicius M, Boddaert N, Belin P, et al. Temporal lobe dysfunction in childhood autism: a PET study. Am J Psychiatry 2000;157:1988–93.
207. Buchsbaum MS, Hollander E, Haznedar MM, et al. Effect of fluoxetine on regional cerebral metabolism in autistic spectrum disorders: a pilot study. Int J Neuropsychopharmacol 2001;4(2):119–25.
208. Nakamura K, Sekine Y, Ouchi Y, et al. Brain serotonin and dopamine transporter bindings in adults with high-functioning autism. Arch Gen Psychiatry 2010;67(1):59–68.

Index

Note: Page numbers of article titles are in **boldface** type.

PET Clin 5 (2010) 243–246
doi:10.1016/S1556-8598(10)00059-3

U

W

Printed and bound by CPI Group (UK) Ltd, Croydon, CR0 4YY
03/10/2024
01040351-0006